PAMELA ALLARDICE

natural remedies
A-Z

D1419658

HarperCollins*Publishers*

NOTE TO THE READER

This book should be regarded as a reference only. You are advised to consult a qualified naturopath, natural therapist or your doctor for treating serious complaints.

HarperCollins*Publishers*

First published in Australia in 1995
Reprinted in 1995

Copyright © Pamela Allardice, 1995

HarperCollins*Publishers*
25 Ryde Road, Pymble, Sydney, NSW 2073, Australia
31 View Road, Glenfield, Auckland 10, New Zealand
77-85 Fulham Palace Road, London W6 8JB, United Kingdom
Hazelton Lanes, 55 Avenue Road, Suite 2900, Toronto, Ontario M5R 3L2
and 1995 Markham Road, Scarborough, Ontario M1B 5M8, Canada
10 East 53rd Street, New York NY 10032, USA

National Library of Australia Cataloguing-in-Publication data:

Allardice, Pamela, 1958–   .
Natural Remedies A–Z.

ISBN 0 7322 5135 4.

1. Naturopathy – Popular works.
2. Therapeutics – Popular works. I. Title.
920.094

Cover design by Cathy Campbell
Printed in Australia by McPherson's Printing Group, Maryborough, Victoria

9 8 7 6 5 4 3 2   95 96 97 98

INTRODUCTION

As more people become concerned with their own health — and specifically with topics such as diet, nutrition, exercise and relaxation — there is an increasing interest in natural remedies and alternative medicine. The natural remedies in this book can all be obtained at health food stores and pharmacies, and, increasingly, you will find them in natural foods sections of supermarkets.

On that first visit to a health food store or pharmacy, the shopper is usually bombarded with information on the latest scientific findings, often in a confusing — and sometimes contradictory — fashion. The situation can be made even more complex when the shopper examines the intriguing and dazzling variety of nutritional supplements for sale, such as vitamins, minerals and strange-sounding herbs. What specific remedies work with particular ailments? And what do all the bewildering terms on the label mean? What are simple and safe remedies you can make yourself at home?

Natural Remedies A-Z is a clear and simple handbook to make sense of the terminology of nutrition and the relationship between nutrition and health. From acidophilus and almonds to yoghurt and zinc, this book gives a clear explanation of over 300 natural remedies, along with a description of their properties and uses.

ACIDOPHILUS

Acidophilus is a special culture, usually made from goat's milk, which will enhance and replace missing intestinal or vaginal flora. (Such a loss is usually triggered by antibiotics, the contraceptive pill or vaginal infections.) A smart preventive move is to take an acidophilus formula — tablet or capsule — orally. Additionally, mix half a teaspoon of acidophilus powder in a glass of warm water and swish this through your mouth, to combat any yeast in the oral cavity, before swallowing it.

Acidophilus-based yoghurt is excellent for use as a gentle low-pressure douche. Buy the natural unsweetened varieties for this purpose or buy a yoghurt starter culture and make your own. An individual already afflicted with candidiasis should eat acidophilus yoghurt every day and douche with the diluted yoghurt.

AGAR

Constipation is an increasing complaint among us today, due largely to the introduction of greater amounts of processed foods into our diet. A powdered seaweed supplement, agar or agar-agar, if added to stewed fruit, is a known remedy for such cases. Being a useful thickener, agar is also often listed as an ingredient in Japanese cookery and recipes based on macrobiotic principles.

Tip:
Agrimony is a useful bath herb, and is particularly recommended for aching muscles and rheumatism.

AGRIMONY

The leaves of agrimony (*Agrimonia eupatoria*) can be bruised and bound onto a sprain. A warm, soothing compress can be made by softening the leaves in a sieve held over boiling water, then pulping them and applying as a poultice (*see also* Arnica). This method is also useful for washing wounds and drawing out splinters.

The crushed roots and leaves of agrimony were once used to make the famous French toilet water, E*au d'Arquebusade*, which was used on wounds caused by hand guns — or *arquebuses* — during days when duels were more common! A tea made from powdered agrimony is said to be useful for gastrointestinal problems, and agrimony sometimes features as an ingredient in products which treat constipation and skin disorders.

ALCOHOL

No smiles, please — I am not advocating this as a 'natural remedy'! Alcohol is, however, mentioned in many of the recipes in this book. As the unlicensed sale of pure alcohol is illegal in most countries, vodka is listed as being a substitute. Alcohol is usually included in both commercial preparations and in the recipes detailed in this book for its preservative properties.

BASIC TOILET WATER

15 ml essential oil of your choice (lavender, rose, bergamot, orange flower and so on)

1 litre ethyl alcohol (or 80 proof vodka)

2 teaspoons rosewater

Mix the oil with the alcohol until well blended; stir in the rosewater. Pour the toilet water into clear, clean glass jars or bottles and cap securely. Allow to mature for 6 to 8 weeks before using; store in refrigerator.

ALDER

The dried bark and leaves of the common alder (A*lnus glutinosa*) are said to be useful when brewed as a tea and given to patients suffering chronic indigestion and dyspepsia. The fresh leaves are mentioned in early herbal texts as being used to prepare soothing poultices for inflamed skin. Alder has household applications, too: a solution made by steeping alder leaves in vinegar may be used as a spray to ward off fleas. A diluted version may be used to deter vermin closer to home, namely as a hair and scalp bath for a child with lice, and to cure scabies.

ALFALFA

Alfalfa (*Medicago sativa*) is also well known as lucerne, and those unfamiliar with natural remedies may wonder why cattle fodder should figure in this book! Alfalfa is rich in vitamins and minerals and the tablets or tea bags you can buy are a worthwhile all-round tonic. For centuries, alfalfa has had a reputation as an 'energising' food for horses — the name comes from the Arab *alfacfacah*, which means 'best feed' — and in ancient Greece and Rome, athletes commenced using alfalfa as a tonic whilst they were in training. Alfalfa sprouts may be easily grown from seed in your garden or just in a jar on the windowsill; they are a healthful and tasty addition to a fresh salad.

ALLSPICE

You probably know the powdered dried berries of the Jamaican pimento or pepper tree (*Pimenta dioica*) better as a flavouring for food. However, the berries of allspice contain an oil that is a natural remedy, too.

This oil may be used in medicines as a digestive, pain reliever and anaesthetic. It is commonly listed as an ingredient in tonics and syrups to treat flatulence, indigestion and diarrhoea, while eugenol (the active chemical agent in allspice oil) is an ingredient in topical preparations for rheumatism and neuralgia, as well as being used as a local anaesthetic by dentists. Allspice oil may be used as an emergency first-aid measure for toothache or, made into a plaster, for neuralgia or headache.

ALMOND OIL

Almond oil is used today in hair conditioners, creams, nail whiteners, polish removers, eye creams, moisturisers, soaps and perfumes. The oil is very fine and penetrating, and is a valuable natural remedy for all dry skin conditions. It may be used externally or internally to 'feed' the skin from within. For dry skin on the feet, wash first with a mixture of 1 tablespoon of bran and 3 tablespoons of strong chamomile infusion (about 6 tablespoons of dried chamomile flowers to 1 cup of water). Rinse, wipe dry and lavish with slightly warmed almond oil.

It is a good idea to regularly apply a warm oil treatment before shampooing, especially for flyaway hair or split ends. Almond oil is one of the best choices, being a very fine oil which will penetrate the hair shaft to moisturise and condition without clogging up the scalp pores. Make a strong herbal oil by bruising a bunch of herbs — chamomile, rosemary and grated burdock are all recommended — and covering them with almond oil. Strain, warm, rub thoroughly into the scalp and hair and wrap tightly in a warm, damp towel. Alternatively, you may add the contents of a vitamin E capsule, or a few drops of rosemary or chamomile essence to the almond oil. Massaging almond oil gently into the scalp to soften it is a useful remedy for an itchy scalp.

Tip:

Chilblains can be very painful. They are often caused by inadequate protection and poor circulation. An excellent year-round habit to get into is hand and finger massage. Firstly, massage each finger from tip to base, then the palm and back of the hand, with warmed almond oil. Then clench your hands and open them. Spread your fingers wide and rotate them slowly.

Wrinkles cannot be avoided but their appearance can be minimised. Gently pat almond oil into those areas where wrinkles first begin to appear — around the nose, mouth and eyes. This will be a great help. Or make your own rich all-over body moisturising cream, based on almond oil, to combat premature wrinkles.

Tip:

Very dry or split nails will revel in a nourishing treat of 2 teaspoons beaten egg yolk, 2 teaspoons almond oil and 2 teaspoons raw honey. Mix and massage a thin film into the nails and leave overnight. To soften the cuticles, use the same mixture, substituting pineapple juice for the honey.

For this, take ¼ cup fine almond oil, ¼ cup rose petals, 3 teaspoons beeswax and ½ cup boiling water. Steep rose petals in boiling water for half an hour. Melt the oil and beeswax together in a double boiler. Strain the rosewater and add the melted wax and oil, stirring constantly. Pour the mixture into a glass jar and refrigerate. After it has set, whip the cream till it is smooth and light. A few drops of rose oil can be substituted for the rosewater.

Here is another recipe which has a delightful aroma and is very good for smoothing on dry problem areas, such as heels and elbows.

Melt ½ cup petroleum jelly with 3 teaspoons almond oil and 1 teaspoon beeswax in a double boiler, then add 3 teaspoons of lanolin. Carefully stir in ¼ cup purified water and cool. Then add ½ teaspoon of vanilla extract and whip until creamy and smooth. Store in the refrigerator in a clean, tightly lidded glass jar.

ALMONDS

One of the most interesting of recent discoveries in the world of natural products and remedies is to do with almonds. It is hypothesised that almonds may be excellent preventives of cancer. A daily intake of even just six may be of great benefit in our diet.

Almonds were prized by the ancient Greeks and

Romans because they were supposed to prevent drunkenness. According to Roman naturalist Pliny the Elder, many notorious wine drinkers avoided intoxication by munching the nuts.

During the Middle Ages, almonds were used extensively for cooking, as medicine and in cosmetics, where their emollient properties make them ideal ingredients. The blanched nuts are also an old folk remedy for heartburn and were used for many disorders, especially those affecting the kidneys, bladder and biliary ducts.

Blanched almonds can be made into meal which is used in confectionery and as a sauce thickener. The meal may also be used as a base for soothing skin-bleaching pastes and cleansing masks. Sometimes it is added to soap.

Making your own almond meal is easy and you'll be less likely to run into problems with rancidity, since whole nuts store better. To blanch the almonds, cover the nuts with boiling water, let stand for 2 minutes, then rub off the brown skin. Dry the nuts and chop them up coarsely. Pulverise them by whirling in a blender at top speed, but add only ¼ cup of the chopped nuts to the blender at a time. Almonds seem to be the only nuts that don't get oily when they're run through the blender.

Almond 'milk', made by blending the meal with water, sugar and acacia gum to make a smooth thick liquid, may be strained and used as a substitute for milk in cooking.

Almond 'butter', available in your health food store and some supermarkets, makes a rich protein substitute for peanut butter, and is usually well tolerated by diabetics.

Almond milk was also once used as a soothing, nourishing skin lotion, and continues to be so used today. In his *Herball*, mediaeval herbalist John Gerard observed that 'oil of almonds makes smooth the hands and face of delicate persons and cleanseth the skin from all spots and pimples'. Make your own almond milk cleanser with the following recipe.

Blanch 225 g almonds and pulverise in a blender. Add 1 egg white, ¼ cup milk, ⅓ cup water and 2 tablespoons vodka to the almond meal and blend together at medium speed. Pour the mixture into a bowl and refrigerate, covered, for 2 hours. Strain through cheese-cloth, then bottle the liquid and refrigerate. Use the almond milk as a morning cleanser, or following the use of a regular cleanser.

ALOE VERA

Aloe vera (*Aloe barbadensis*) is a member of the lily family. Its thick, sappy pulp has remarkable antiseptic and heal-ing properties and promotes the growth of healthy skin cells. A great healer for skin eruptions is straight aloe vera pulp: just snap a leaf open and apply. Also, pure aloe vera can help get rid of blemishes without scarring. Saturate a cotton pad and smooth the cooling gel onto the affected area. (It is, incidentally, very easy to grow as a house plant. Try placing one in your kitchen — then the marvellous healing gel is close by to treat any burn or cut.)

Tip:

For roughened, work-stained hands, wash your hands well in lukewarm water, dry, and massage lavishly with aloe vera gel before pulling on cotton gloves and going to bed.

Stabilised aloe gel is available in bottled form and this may be added to your current creams and shampoos or slathered, neat, onto sun-burned or dry skin. Aloe vera powder, gel and concentrate are all to be found listed as ingre-dients of natural beauty products. A marvellous firming mask can be made by combining raw egg white and aloe gel. Follow this with a moisturising treatment.

Aloe vera has several proven benefits for hair, helping to tighten the outer layer on each strand of hair, making it smooth in appearance and better able to reflect light — in short, making it shinier. This produces tangle-free tresses that shine with health. Aloe's antiseptic action also works for dandruff and other scalp problems.

ANGELICA

John Parkinson in his *The Theatre of Plantes* (1640) wrote that 'the whole plante, both leafe, roote and seede, is of an excellent comfortable scent, savour and taste', adding, cryptically, that a powder made from the dried roots 'will abate the rage of lust in young persons'. In very early times, angelica (*Angelica archangelica*) was thought to be an anti-witch herb, and both the seeds and musky gum from the stems were used in potions to safeguard property and persons. According to tradition, angelica's medicinal prowess and ability to ward off pestilence were revealed to humans by the angels, hence the name. During the Great Plague of London in 1664–65, dried and powdered angelica root was mixed with vinegar and used to wash clothes and linen. The seeds were burned in chafing dishes to perfume and fumigate houses.

Angelica remains an important herb for use in natural remedies. It is probably best known as a digestive and demulcent, being often prescribed by herbalists for patients recuperating from a gastrointestinal illness, or as a tea for small children who cannot tolerate heavy food after sickness. The stalks may be blanched and eaten rather like celery, or candied and used as a decoration. The aromatic oil distilled from the seeds and roots of angelica is restorative and soothing to the nerves and may be used in inhalations to induce sleep.

ANISEED

In earlier times, aniseed (*Pimpinella anisum*) was considered so valuable it was used as 'money' to pay taxes. Today, it is better known as a common flavouring, familiar to all cooks. But did you know a teaspoon of the seeds, steeped in 600 ml of boiling water and then cooled, is an excellent natural remedy for colic in babies? The essential oil may be used externally, or taken internally as a tea, to relieve cramping and spasms such as those due to menstruation: a few drops in a mug of hot water are all you need.

Tip:
Essential oil of aniseed is a stimulating and strongly aromatic scent and is often included in products such as aftershave for men.

Aniseed oil is also used widely in cough lozenges and syrups. An infusion of aniseed will make a cleansing and refreshing mouthwash or gargle. Alternatively, add 3 to 4 drops of the essential oil to 250 ml of cooled boiled water. This can also be used after tooth extraction to reduce swelling and bleeding.

ANTIOXIDANTS

High-dose combinations of the antioxidant vitamins A and C and zinc, as well as topical applications of vitamin E, are the hallmark of today's preventive dermatology (*see also Vitamins and Zinc*).

Clinical tests prove these nutrients are particularly important in the treatment of contact rashes and dermatitis; similarly, pruritic skin conditions frequently respond to an appropriate intake of vitamins A and C. Athlete's foot and other fungal infections respond well to topical vitamin E and oral intake of the antioxidant vitamins, as do dandruff, cracked skin between the fingers and toes and stretch marks. Antioxidant vitamin supplements help the body to strengthen its defence system, thus reducing the chance of reinfection, and to heal damaged skin tissue.

APPLES

Apple water is excellent for feverish patients. Prepare it by slicing three washed, unpeeled apples. Simmer until they are soft. Strain the apples, add a piece of lemon for flavour and chill before drinking.

Fresh apple juice is a little-known cosmetic, having excellent restorative and tonic properties for the skin. Peel and core one small apple, process in a blender until you have a liquid, and then put through a sieve. Combine this with 1 tablespoon of whole milk and enough fuller's earth to thicken (approximately 1 tablespoon) and use as a cleansing mask for dull or scaly skin. Rinse off and tone and moisturise as usual.

Another idea is to cook the apple flesh and combine with equal parts of cream, honey and ground oatmeal to make a rich and nourishing facial mask. Warm slightly and spread over your face.

APRICOT KERNEL OIL

Cold-pressed apricot kernel oil is rich in vitamin E and makes a splendid massage treatment. Smooth over the throat and chest with light, upward strokes and dab onto crepey skin around the eyes to prevent further dryness and wrinkling. For best results, warm oil first and 'iron' skin smooth with a spoon.

Use this time-honoured treatment in your hair, too, to replace oils lost by vigorous and overregular shampooing, and to protect your hair by coating each shaft and reducing moisture loss. Warm a little apricot kernel oil and massage into your hair. Wrap a hot, damp towel around your head and leave on for an hour. If you can reheat the towel occasionally, so much the better. Shampoo (it may take more than one lathering to get the oil out) and finish with a cream rinse or conditioner.

Tip:

If you are running, jogging or playing winter sports, apply a thin film of apricot kernel oil to skin to protect against chafing.

APRICOT KERNELS

The finely ground kernels from the apricot fruit are sometimes included as an ingredient in natural cosmetics, notably body and face exfoliants. They have a gentle anti-scurf action, helping to remove dead skin cells and oils from the body; commercial products, by way of comparison, usually use finely milled plastic beads.

ARNICA

Arnica (*Arnica montana*) is a remarkable herbal remedy. Father John Kunzle, a great herbalist of the 19th century, recommended that it be made into an ointment or tincture for use 'in the case of sprains, dislocations and swellings caused by them'. This is still good advice. Arnica tinctures (sometimes called arnica extract) and arnica ointments can be used as a natural remedy for bruises, sprains, swellings and common athletic injuries. You can make your own arnica tincture by soaking a handful of fresh arnica flowers in pure alcohol (or 80 proof vodka) for 2 weeks.

To make an arnica compress for sprains or bruises, add 1 tablespoon of arnica tincture to cold water and mix; wet a towel with the mixture and apply to the injured area. Remember, however, that arnica is never to be used on open wounds, only on unbroken skin.

ARROWROOT

Arrowroot (*Maranta arundinacea*) is a demulcent, nutritious powdered starch obtained from the dried rhizomes of a West Indian plant. It is nonirritating and a great nutritive — because of this, it is well suited as a natural remedy for infants and convalescents. Boil 2 or 3 tablespoons in 250 ml of water and season to taste with honey or lemon juice. This can be drunk or added to fruit-based jellies or puddings. Arrowroot is also used as a thickening agent in cosmetics and various cream preparations; it is very soothing to the skin, particularly when made into a gel.

ARTICHOKE

For severe eczema, Maurice Messegue's recipe for 'hand and skin baths' works as well today as it did in the 18th century and is a positive alternative to topical cortisone treatments. Steep artichoke leaves in sufficient hot water to cover and allow to cool; strain. Then soak the affected area in the 'artichoke water' for 10 minutes at a time.

AVOCADO OIL

Pure cold-pressed avocado oil is a rich source of vitamin D and is a palatable alternative to cod liver oil, should you wish to take a spoonful each day. It is an excellent treatment for all dry skin conditions. It is also excellent for brittle and dry hair. Mash a whole avocado, massage into hair and scalp, cover with a plastic bag and leave for an hour before shampooing.

An old-fashioned preventive treatment for wrinkles is to soak in a hot bath and apply avocado oil generously over the face and neck, paying particular attention to dry areas around the lips and eyes. The steam from the bath encourages the oil to sink into the skin. The insides of avocado skins are also very good for cleaning and softening skin. Try the following anti-ageing remedy.

Avocado and Honey Beauty Drops

1 egg

2 tablespoons avocado oil

2 tablespoons raw honey

Separate the egg and process the yolk, oil and honey in a blender. When the mixture thickens, add the egg white and blend till smooth. Apply a few drops to the eyelids. Smooth into the area around the eyes, rest the eyes for 20 minutes and then rinse off. Apply twice daily.

BALM

See Lemon balm.

BARBERRY

This plant is closely related to the Oregon grape (*Mahonia aquifolium*), which is used by herbalists to stimulate the immune system naturally. Barberry (*Berberis vulgaris*) is an ornamental shrub which has been known to herbal healers as a natural antibiotic for many centuries. Gardeners may know it better as sowberry or jaundice berry, a reference to both its red berries and yellow flowers. In very small doses, a tincture of barberry may be prescribed by a natural therapist to treat liver conditions and gastric upsets, while the bark may be used to brew a tea which will help counter gingivitis and other oral hygiene conditions.

Today, however, its most exciting implication to the world of natural remedies is its antibiotic capacity — the essential oil, berberine, found in the berries has quite remarkable powers for fighting micro-organisms in the body; it has been successfully tested as a remedy for dysentery and diarrhoea. It should only be taken according to a qualified herbalist's instructions, however, as a too-large dose can actually cause diarrhoea.

BARLEY

Barley (*Hordeum vulgare*) water has been used from earliest times to assist patients in high fever. Because it has no irritating properties, it is especially helpful where either the chest lining or intestinal lining is inflamed, such as will occur with a severe bout of gastrointestinal flu. Children suffering from diarrhoea and bowel inflammations will also benefit from barley water. Barley water and barley 'milk' (made by simmering barley in skim milk or soy milk for 15 minutes, then straining and cooling) form a very soothing mix for a patient recuperating from intestinal problems, once the vomiting stage has passed.

A refreshing and nutritious drink may be made from the juice of young barley plants, which contain an extraordinary range of nutrients, including vitamins B_1, B_2, B_6, E and C, high levels of betacarotene (the precursor to vitamin A), pantothenic acid and folic acid, plus the minerals calcium, magnesium, potassium, iron, selenium and zinc.

BASIL

Seventeenth century herbalist Jacques Tournefort was convinced that smelling basil (*Ocimum basilicum*) would cause venomous scorpions to breed in a patient's brain and this story meant — understandably — that basil was viewed askance by physicians for some time. Despite this, basil has been widely used as a medicinal herb, usually in tea or essential oil form, primarily as a digestive aid for settling an upset stomach and allaying nausea. John Gerard recommended basil 'to procure a cheerful and merrie heart', which was presumably a reference to its invigorating and tonic effects.

Tip:
Keeping a pot of basil on a windowsill will deter flies.

Dried basil leaves were once used as snuff. Essential oil of basil, rubbed on the temples, is said to cure a headache. Both the oil and the fresh or dried leaves may be steeped in pure boiled or spring water to make a lotion to cleanse and tone the complexion. Modern research confirms that this can even help acne sufferers, for basil kills bacteria on the skin. In the Philippines and South America, basil is used to get rid of intestinal worms and also, in poultice form, to treat ringworm. Possibly due to its association with aphrodisiacs, basil tea is still used in some countries to supposedly assist labour.

BATH MITTS

Bath mitts are only now getting some highly deserved attention as natural beauty aids. They're a great way to get the concentrated power of herbs to where they're most needed — on your skin! They are easy to make: simply stitch three layers of fabric together on three sides (face cloths work well for this, or use any natural absorbent fabric — silk feels wonderful!). The open end now forms two pockets, one for your hand and one to hold those magical herbs. Try this recipe for dry, itchy skin.

HERBAL CLEANSER

60 g cornstarch

60 g almond meal

60 g oatmeal

60 g cornmeal

30 g dried chamomile flowers

Spray with essential oil if extra fragrance is desired.

BATHS

You can buy most of the herbs needed for a naturally healing and beautifying bath from your health food store. Make a full bath infusion by pouring boiling water onto dried herbs, steeping them and then adding the cooled liquid to the bathwater. Alternatively, pack the herbs into bath bags and suspend under the tap whilst the hot water is running.

For a calming bath to comfort aching limbs, combine bay leaves, chamomile, lemon balm and lime flowers. Rosemary is also excellent for relieving stiff joints and relaxing aching muscles; it was used by Roman soldiers to relieve their tired feet after a long march. An infusion of birch bark is an ancient remedy for soothing aches in muscles and joints. It may be used after exercising, or for the discomfort of arthritis.

For a refreshing, invigorating bath, lavender and eucalyptus have a brisk scent and are both natural disinfectants. Borage, sage and peppermint are all enlivening herbs. Spearmint is a tonic for body and soul: try a spearmint bath for a wonderful start to the day!

Other sweet-smelling herbs which can be blended in any combination to your personal taste, and have a mildly tonic effect in the bath, are marjoram, basil, meadowsweet, and pennyroyal. Try this recipe for a scented bath: combine equal quantities of rose petals, chamomile flowers, orange and lemon flowers and leaves, and orange and lemon peel. Simmer all together in a muslin bag in water and add the liquid to the bath. Then use the bag as a body scrub.

Packs of dried elder flowers and leaves are usually for sale in health food stores. Use them in a bath bag, to which you have also added equal quantities of chopped geranium root and nettle leaves, to help heal minor irritations of the skin. Dried marigold flowers will aid chafed and dry skin.

To warm up quickly after a cold autumn day, use this recipe which promotes circulation and softens the skin: steep 15 g of fresh grated ginger in boiling water, mix the liquid with witch hazel and a little almond oil and rub briskly into wet skin whilst in the bath, using a loofah or body brush. Crushed cloves and bay leaves are also an excellent combination for a warming winter bath.

When making up your mixtures, add a tablespoon of fine oatmeal or bran — they have an extra-cleansing effect and will leave the skin especially silky and smooth. Lovage can also be added. It is a natural deodorant and has a pleasing smell of its own.

Take the time whenever the mood strikes to enjoy a

bath. Remember, you are pampering and caring for the most important asset you possess — your healthy, happy body.

BATH SALTS

Bath salts are easily made and can be stored indefinitely. They're toning and most refreshing. Spray three parts sea salt, one part powdered Irish moss and one part bicarbonate of soda with a fragrant essential oil and toss well. If you would like to add colour to your salt mixture, spray with a few drops of pure vegetable dye and mix well.

BAY

Bay (*Laurus nobilis*) leaves, berries and bark have all been used medicinally since very early times. The pungent smell was thought to repel infection, so physicians would rub their hands with the crushed leaves after ministering to a sick patient, in the belief that this would protect them. During outbreaks of plague, residents of ancient Rome were advised to burn bay trees in public places.

This herb is usually available in essential oil form, or the dried berries and leaves may be burned in incense, added to potpourri, steeped in a tea for a bath additive or, of course, used in cookery. Aromatic bay oil has long been used as a soothing rub for bruises and aching joints due to arthritis and rheumatism, with 17th century herbalist Nicolas Culpeper recommending it for 'all griefes of the jointes', and it is still a popular natural remedy for sprains.

An inhalation may be used to clear a headache due to blocked nasal passages. It was once thought to be a cure for colic; however, it is not now recommended that bay

Tip:

Keeping a few dried bay leaves in your kitchen canisters will repel moths and weevils crushed bay leaves in cupboards will also send cockroaches scurrying.

oil be given to children under two years of age. One of the more intriguing findings in herbal medicine research points to the use of oil of bay in stress management, for the scent has been shown to actually lower blood pressure and induce feelings of relaxation.

BAYBERRY

Also called waxberry, candleberry or wax myrtle, bayberry (*Myrica cerifera*) is probably better known to herbalists than the general public for the astringent and tonic effects of its root bark. It is native to the woods and marshes of northern America and was first used medicinally by the Choctaw tribe of Native Americans, who boiled the leaves and drank the resulting tea as a treatment for fever. The root bark is high in volatile tannins and resins which make it a valuable treatment for any conditions which involve inflammation or infection of the bowels; similarly, it may be prescribed by a natural therapist to a patient who is troubled with excessive menstrual bleeding and/or uterine discharge. It may also be used as a gargle for throat infections and a herbalist may use bayberry tincture to treat slow-healing wounds because of its astringent effect.

Most recently, bayberry has made somewhat of a comeback in more generally available products, and you may find it included in remedies for diarrhoea; interestingly, modern research has not only confirmed its ability to treat looseness of the bowels, but has also identified an antibiotic chemical that is contained in the root bark, myricitrin, which helps to fight dangerous bacteria which could be causing the bowel problem in the first place. Bayberry should only be used with the approval of your natural therapist and/or doctor as it can be contra-indicated for people with high blood pressure or circulatory disorders.

BEANS

Beans or pulses come in a great many more varieties than just the common-and-garden string bean or French bean (*Phaseolus vulgaris*). Other beans you may become familiar with include the Adzuki (a small, sweet bean used in Asian puddings and savoury foods); the broad bean (actually the ripe seed of *Vicia faba*); the butter bean (the seed of *Phaseolus lunatus*); the haricot or red kidney bean (the ripe seed of *Phaseolus vulgaris* — this is the bean used for making baked beans and the one most likely to cause undesirable windy side effects); the locust bean (the seed of *Ceratonia siliqua*); the mung or green gram bean (mainly used for its sprouts); the runner bean (the seed of *Phaseolus multiflorus*, always eaten unripe in the green pod) and the scarlet runner bean (the seed of *Phaseolus coccineus*, always eaten sliced in the green pod). You may also come across other dried beans, such as lentils (often eaten with wheat and peas in Middle Eastern diets) and garbanzos or chickpeas (hummus and falafel are two foods based on the chickpea). Pintos and black beans, more common in Latin American cuisine, are also worth experimenting with.

Fresh beans and bean pods are usually higher in vitamins A and C than the dried varieties; they are also good sources of folic acid, B vitamins and iron. Fresh beans may be eaten steamed or cooked by themselves or with other vegetables. They also have a diuretic action and bean pod tea is useful for treating kidney or bladder disorders. There is also a homoeopathic bean tincture, which may be bought or prescribed for treating rheumatism. All the dried beans or legumes represent a very important 'natural remedy' for our Western diet today — in short, when we are looking for foods which are lower in fat, lower in salt and lower in calories (not to mention lower in cost), legumes are one of the best substitutes for meat and fat-laden dishes we can find. You may also come across finely ground dried 'bean meal' in some health food stores: this may be used in much the same way as cornflour, to treat itching, reddened or inflamed skin. It appears to be particularly beneficial as a soothing dressing for acneous conditions.

BEESWAX

This is listed as an ingredient in nearly all natural cosmetics you will see for sale. It is primarily included for its nourishing and emollient properties. It is also traditionally used as an emulsifier and a binder in all manner of cosmetic creams, notably lip salves and protectives. If you wish to use beeswax in any of the recipes mentioned in this book, you will usually be able to purchase it from either pharmacies or hobby shops; it is generally sold in pressed cakes.

BASIC COSMETIC CREAM

½ cup grated beeswax

½ cup almond oil

4 tablespoons distilled water

a few drops of essential oil, to preference

Melt the wax in a double boiler over low heat. Add the oil and beat very slowly, then add water, continuing to beat until the mixture starts to emulsify. Remove from the heat and allow to cool slightly, adding fragrant oil if desired. Continue to whisk until all is thoroughly blended, then pour into clean glass jars and cap securely.

BENZOIN

Also known as 'gum benjamin' or benzoin simplex, this is a type of resin derived from the reddish-brown aromatic balsam of a Javanese tree. It is often listed as an ingredient in all sorts of natural remedies, from tonics and tinctures to beauty preparations. The Arabs are believed to have been the first to use benzoin as a cosmetic. It is primarily included for its preservative properties; it is also a powerful astringent and has the effect of emulsifying wool fat (lanolin). If you are going to make a recipe which refers to benzoin, you will usually be able to purchase it from a pharmacy, either in powder or tincture form.

BETONY

Betony (Betonica officinalis) is a perennial herb, and a member of the Labiatae family; it is native to Britain and Europe and is often to be seen near old churches and monuments, having been planted many centuries ago as a means of warding away evil spirits and witches. (This was, interestingly, the case with quite a few medicinal herbs — once their benefits to health were identified, it was assumed, by association, that they were 'magical' or, in some way, a gift from heaven.)

Modern herbalists may prescribe betony tea, usually based on a dosage of 1 to 3 g of the dried herb three times a day, as a natural remedy for migraines and digestive upsets such as diarrhoea. It acts as a tonic and stimulant to the cerebral and head area as well as a stimulant to the digestive system. Betony tea may also be prescribed for asthmatics and as a tonic for patients suffering catarrhal congestion and associated gastritis. The old 'herb wyfes' used to say it helped children who were not growing as strongly as they should, and it is still a useful natural remedy for general debility. You may also see betony listed as an ingredient in herbal ointments for cuts and sores because of its astringent and stimulating effects. Do not take betony tea without the advice of your herbalist or a responsible natural therapist, as too much will cause vomiting.

BIOFLAVONOIDS

This complex, sometimes incorrectly called vitamin P, is complementary to vitamin C. In fact, there is now much evidence to suggest that the utilisation of vitamin C in the body is enhanced by the presence of the bioflavonoids, including rutin and hesperidin. Many vitamin C supplements contain added bioflavonoids for this reason.

Bioflavonoids help to strengthen the capillary walls and veins and are therefore important in the treatment of unattractive surface capillaries and other related varicose conditions. Inflamed and painful gums which bleed easily can be improved by adopting a citrus-rich diet, for the bioflavonoids found in orange or lemon pith help strengthen these tiny capillaries. Other good food sources include rosehips, capsicums and other citrus fruits such as grapefruit and limes. Some results of deficiency to watch for are dermatitis, fatigue and muscular weakness.

BIOTIN

A member of the vitamin B family, biotin has been advertised as a cure for certain types of baldness when included in natural hair care products. Indeed, it may improve dermatitis, dandruff, hair loss and seborrhoea. Results of dietary biotin deficiency include nervousness, dermatitis, dandruff and hair loss. A deficiency of biotin can also cause depression, muscle pain and drowsiness. Good food sources include brewer's yeast, brown rice, soya beans, liver and kidney.

BIRCH

Birch (*Betula alba*) bark is an ancient remedy for soothing aches in muscles or joints. It is often listed as an ingredient in rubs and liniments for sports enthusiasts and for treating the discomfort of arthritis and rheumatism. The leaves and bark can both be made into a natural remedy for arthritis and rheumatism pain. To make your own, take 4 handfuls of silver birch bark and steep in enough water to cover in a non-aluminium saucepan over low to medium heat for at least 30 minutes. Strain through a nonmetallic sieve and add to warm bathwater. This recipe may also be used for a footbath. A tea made from the leaves may be used to relieve gout and is also useful for kidney and bladder stones, and diarrhoea.

Tip:

An infusion of birch bark has been used since very early times as a natural remedy for skin irritations. It is a naturally astringent and healing herb.

BLACKBERRY

Blackberry (*Rubus fruticosus*) wine was once very popular, both as a medicine and as a cordial. Greek and Roman physicians often referred to wild blackberries in their journals and writings. Pliny the Elder tells us, in his *Natural History*, that 'The berries have a desiccative and astringent virtue and are a most appropriate remedy for the gums and inflammations of the tonsils'.

Another reference to blackberries' health-giving properties comes from herbalist John Gerard, who in 1597 wrote about the leaves: 'The young buds or tender tops of the Bramble Bush, the flowers, the leaves and the unripe fruit, do very much dry and binde withall: being chewed they take away the heate and inflammations of the mouths and almonds of the throte. They heale the eyes that hang out. The leaves of the Bramble boiled in water with honie, allum and a little white wine added thereto, maketh a most excellent lotion or washing water, to heale the sores of the mouth and fastneth the teeth.'

Interestingly, modern-day herbalists still consider blackberries and their juice to be very useful as natural remedies for treating mouth infections and for soothing redness or inflammation of the eyes caused by allergic reactions or strain. As is the case with several other berries, notably strawberries (*see Strawberries*), an infusion of blackberry leaves has been used to help treat diarrhoea.

An infusion of the root has similar astringent properties and may be used either internally to help control gastrointestinal upsets or externally as a bath tonic to freshen and clarify the skin. Blackberry leaves were always included in old-time recipes for baths 'to be taken in spring' to rejuvenate the body, sluggish after winter. The berries while not being valuable medicinally are nonetheless a rich source of vitamins and some minerals. They are particularly high in vitamin C and thiamine and contain some calcium, iron, potassium, riboflavin and niacin as well.

BLACK COHOSH

Black cohosh (*Cimicifuga racemosa*) or black snakeroot was well known by the Native Americans as a natural remedy for gynaecological complaints and during childbirth. It is interesting to learn that black cohosh was also one of the main ingredients in the famous 19th century patent medicine, 'Lydia Pinkham's Female Compound'. In those days, they claimed it was good for treating 'hysterical' complaints, meaning female ailments like menstrual pain and cramping.

Black cohosh has strong antispasmodic, sedative and oestrogenic effects, making it very useful in the treatment of any inflammatory condition associated with spasm or tension, such as dysmenorrhoea or menstrual pain. It is usually prescribed by a herbalist in the form of a tea. In small quantities, it may be found as an ingredient in women's health or 'PMT' formulas for menstrual discomfort; it is now also being prescribed to treat menopausal discomfort, high blood pressure and muscular rheumatism. However, it should really only be taken under the direction of a doctor and/or natural therapist, and it must not be used during pregnancy.

BLACKCURRANT

In Russia, blackcurrants (*Ribes nigrum*) were always an important crop and were harvested for wine making as well as for medicinal use. There are some references to blackcurrants being preserved in whisky in Ireland and used as a 'cough punch'. One of the earliest references is in the 1579 *Historie of Plantes* by Ram Dodoen. From that time, blackcurrants really came into their own, being made up into a wide variety of preserves, jams, jellies and cordials. Cooks found that they were admirable for their 'jelling' qualities, being a good source of pectin and therefore setting without too much effort.

Once the blackcurrant became cultivated for culinary use, its medicinal qualities became highly regarded as well. In 1779, John Abercrombie recommended that a few blackcurrant bushes be planted in all gardens 'for wholesome medicinal use'. Most often, blackcurrants were boiled down with sugar and made into a 'rob' or syrup for use as a gargle or cough medicine. An old country name for blackcurrants was 'Squinancy berries', a corruption of 'quinsy', which is an old name for a form of tonsillitis.

These medicinal benefits of blackcurrants should not surprise us. The fruit is fairly bursting with vitamin C — in fact, blackcurrants contain more vitamin C than do oranges, making the juice and syrup very effective in the treatment of sore throats, fevers, coughs and colds, as well as tonsillitis. Blackcurrant juice or cordial also tends to be better tolerated by a small, sick child than the more acid orange juice. Blackcurrants are an excellent source of thiamine, riboflavin and niacin, as well as a fair source of the minerals calcium, potassium and phosphorus. The latter nutrient is especially beneficial for recuperating patients as it helps to replenish tissue salts and fluid lost during bouts of vomiting or diarrhoea.

BLACK HAW

Probably better known as sweet viburnum (*Viburnum prunifolium*), this is another 'woman's herb'. The bark has long been used to brew a tea to treat gynaecological disorders. In appropriate doses — approximately 2 g of the dried bark up to three times per day — it is a valuable and effective natural remedy for excessive menstrual flow and menstrual cramping or pain, having a powerful astringent and antispasmodic effect on the female reproductive system.

Traditionally, it has been used as a uterine relaxant, meaning that at one level of dosage it can prevent threatened miscarriage due to an irritable womb; however, an excess can actually bring on a miscarriage. The herb itself is readily available throughout the world and, at the appropriate dosage, is a boon to women who might otherwise be incapacitated for a number of days each month due to excessive menstrual flow; however, it should only be used in medicinal amounts, and in consultation with your doctor and/or natural therapist.

BLUEBERRY

Blueberries (*Vaccinium* spp.) were once used medicinally in tonics for treating coughs and head colds. As long ago as the 17th century, herbalist Nicolas Culpeper was recommending that 'The juice of the berries [be] made into a syrup, or the pulp made into a conserve with sugar. Drink up to 2 or 3 cups a day.' This still makes good natural health sense, for as with most berries, blueberries are a good source of vitamin C and iron, along with calcium, phosphorus, magnesium and potassium; they are naturally low in sodium and sugar.

BONESET

This oddly named herb, more correctly known as *Eupatorium perfoliatum*, does not, in fact, knit bones back together. Its name came about as a result of its use in treating what used to be known as 'bone-break fever', or dengue fever. It was also known as feverwort for this reason, and has been traditionally used to treat arthritis and other conditions worsened by damp, such as night sweats, colds and constipation.

Boneset is a perennial herb, somewhat reminiscent of yarrow in appearance, and its leaves and flower tops are used to manage fever, usually in tea form (approximately 1 to 3 g of the dried herb up to three times per day). This herb is especially useful for respiratory-associated fevers, such as flu and catarrhal conditions, helping to 'diffuse' the fever from the body. Herbalists have been known to call it 'the herbal aspirin', and in Germany, where herbal medicine is more widely accepted than it is here as yet, it is readily prescribed for colds and flu.

BORAGE

The leaves and flowers of borage (*Borago officinalis*), or 'the herb of gladness', were once believed to impart bravery. (In fact, its name is thought to have come from the old Celtic *borrach*, meaning 'courage'.) Borage tea was drunk by knights before they competed in jousts and their ladies

Tip:

Borage is a useful natural remedy for inflamed or blood-shot eyes. Make an infusion of borage (1 teaspoon of the dried herb or 1 tablespoon of the fresh to a cup of water) and steep for 5 minutes. Allow to cool slightly, strain, and dip clean cotton wool balls in the infusion, then apply to closed eyes for 10 to 15 minutes. This will have a marked cooling and soothing effect.

would give them kerchiefs embroidered with the blue flowers for luck. Dr Fernie in his *Herbal Simples* (1895) attributed borage's invigorating effect to the fact that 'the fresh juice contains 30 per cent nitrate of potash'.

The fresh leaves and flowers may be used for culinary purposes, and also to make a refreshing and uplifting tea, particularly useful in cases of mild depression. An infusion of the leaves is softening and cleansing for the skin. Borage is a good general blood purifier, meaning it encourages the clearing away of toxic residues from the tissues via the bloodstream. To make a tonic tea, infuse a tablespoon of the chopped fresh leaves in a cup of boiling water for 10 to 15 minutes; strain and drink.

BORAX

This is a mineral salt, often included in natural cosmetics and creams for its antiseptic properties. It has a slightly acidic effect, and is used by cosmetic chemists to emulsify beeswax in their preparation of a base for a cream or lotion. You can use it to make a simple and soothing-to-the-skin bath additive.

Tip:

Experiment with using other dry ingredients, too, such as soap flakes, almond meal or orrisroot powder, for their additional cleansing or cosmetic properties.

BASIC BATH SALTS

¾ cup borax

1 to 2 teaspoons essential oil of your choice

(eucalyptus, lavender, jasmine and so on)

Combine oil with borax in a lidded container. Use a heaped teaspoon per bath.

BRAN

Over the past few years bran has become a most popular food supplement and natural remedy, with even the most conservative of doctors now recommending it for a variety of bowel disorders. Why the sudden interest? Is its new-found reputation deserved? And what is bran anyway?

To start with, bran is the high-fibre fraction of whole-wheat which is usually lost in the milling process, a casualty of the processed foods industry. In other words, bran is a substance we would be getting quite naturally if our food-processing techniques were different.

Many research groups have studied the effect of bran on bowel disorders, but perhaps the most decisive work was carried out at Sheffield in England in 1986 when a group of surgeons proved bran was the most effective of several options — including drugs and surgery — for treating the early stages of diverticulitis. Bran also offers benefits for those trying to lose weight. Fewer calories are absorbed from food containing bran, which offers a simple way for weight watchers to minimise their calorie assimilation.

There is much more to the fibre story than just bran, however. The modern diet of a high intake of meat and processed carbohydrates, linked with a low intake of boiled vegetables and fruit, drastically reduces the fibre content within the intestines. The result is slow transit time of the faecal matter, sluggish assimilation, and an inevitable build-up of toxic material. Though we cannot digest fibre, it is absolutely essential for our health and inner cleanliness. The more wholegrain products, raw vegetables and fruit we eat (some with *every* meal), the greater our natural protection and level of health.

BROOM

The tips of broom (*Sarothamnus scoparius*) were once used in herbal medicine, an infusion being considered a cure for dropsy. John Gerard, in his *Herball* of 1597, said 'That worthy Prince of famous memory, Henry VIII of England, was wont to drink the distilled water of Broom-flowers against surfeits and diseases thereof arising'. Unopened broom buds were pickled in brine and used in much the same way as capers are used today.

Modern herbalism has identified broom as a useful natural remedy for palpitations and arrhythmias associated with problems of low blood pressure; it has vasoconstrictive and cardioactive effects, and also acts as a diuretic. It may be used to treat oedema and heart conditions, but must only be used with professional advice.

BUCKWHEAT

Buckwheat is not really a wheat, but a seed. You may be aware of the popular East European dish *kasha*, and this is made from mashed buckwheat. Buckwheat is a particularly healthful food, containing about 15 per cent protein, a good amount of fibre and lots of potassium. Most interestingly, it contains a good deal of rutin (*see* B*ioflavonoids*) and is, in fact, the commercial source for vitamin tablets and capsules containing this nutrient.

Rutin is helpful in strengthening and toning the tiny blood vessels in the body and is used clinically for treating high blood pressure and hardening of the arteries. It is worthwhile getting to know some of the delicious recipes for buckwheat (for example, patties and pancakes) if you are prone to chilblains or capillary fragility. Interestingly, writers such as Leslie Kenton have referred to rutin's stimulant effects on the brainwaves, even in relatively small amounts. It is thought to lift depression as a result.

BURDOCK

The roots and leaves of burdock (*Arctium lappa*) may be used for their medicinal soothing and demulcent effects, both internally as a medicine and externally for skin and hair care. Burdock leaf tea cleanses the system and helps give the hair additional shine from within. It may be used as a cleansing after-shampoo hair rinse, also, to remove last traces of soap and conditioner. The root is often used cosmetically, being soothing and cleansing to irritated skin when used in the bath, or for hair preparations. A tea made from the root and leaves may be taken to treat liver and stomach complaints, having a blood-cleansing and diuretic effect which helps cleanse the system of toxins. The pulped fresh leaves are a valuable natural remedy for swellings, bruises and sprains, for eczema and sores of many kinds, and for bringing down the fever of a patient.

Burdock leaves may be used to treat acne with considerable success. Simmer a handful of burdock leaves in enough water to cover for 5 minutes, then strain. Dip a clean gauze pad or face cloth into the burdock tea and use to wash the affected area of skin. Double the potency of the tea, and it may be used as a tonic and cleansing facial steam for the same problem.

Tip:

Blackheads can be a problem even on a relatively unblemished skin. Excessive pressure may cause local skin damage and the formation of spots or pimples. If this happens, add 50 g of burdock root to 600 ml of cold water. Bring to the boil and simmer for 15 minutes. Allow to cool, strain and apply as a wash to the infected area.

BUTTERMILK

This product is a by-product of butter making. It is soothing and slightly acid, and has an astringent effect on the skin and therefore helps reduce oversized pores. Buttermilk was a very popular old-time natural remedy for freckles, skin discolouration, sunburn, pimples and allergies, and I know several beauty therapists today who still recommend it. Put it on your face with your hands or with cotton wool balls. Let it dry for 10 minutes or so, and then rinse off with tepid water and pat dry with a soft towel. It is a particularly soothing natural remedy to remember in summer, when the skin may be inflamed, or burned by sun or wind, and require cooling.

CABBAGE

Arnica and potato poultices are both remarkable bruise remedies (*see* Arnica and Potato). However, in their absence, if your vegetable drawer yields a cabbage, break the ridges of the large outer leaves, dip briefly into boiling water to soften, and apply to the bruise to reduce swelling. New mothers take note: chilled cabbage leaves are a remarkable remedy for engorged breasts and sore nipples following the birth of a baby. Replace leaves as they assume body heat with freshly chilled ones inside your bra.

Tip:
Cabbage leaves may also be used to prepare a simple facial. Extract the juice from young green leaves and heat slightly; soak gauze pads in the juice and apply to clean and slightly damp skin. Lie back and allow the pads to remain on the skin for 7 to 10 minutes, then remove and rinse face, pat dry.

CALCIUM

This mineral is crucial to the strengthening of bones and teeth and for the transport of other nutrients into individual cells. Healthy teeth need peak nutrition. Calcium is probably the best known supplement, though it is magnesium which results in the formation of decay-resistant enamel. Remember that regular short sunbaths (no more than 15 minutes at a time and never in the middle of the day) are essential for calcium to be correctly absorbed by the body. Good food sources of calcium are milk, cheese, molasses, yoghurt and almonds. Signs of a possible deficiency include acne, eczema, cold sores, excessive perspiration and itchiness.

Tip:
Calcium helps prevent acne. Sunflower seeds are a good source and so are bonemeal supplements.

CALENDULA (MARIGOLD)

The flowers of the marigold (*Calendula officinalis*) were once believed to relieve the pain of a sting from a wasp or bee. Similarly, many herbalists today will use an infusion or tincture of the flowers and buds to treat rashes or recurring sores, and to promote healing and relieve infected insect bites, thus reducing scarring. It is also an excellent styptic for shaving nicks, explaining why marigold or calendula oil or essence is often listed as an ingredient in natural beauty preparations, particularly hand and body lotions, burn ointments and babies' nappy rash creams, usually in conjunction with the skin-healing nutrient, vitamin E.

Marigold vinegar is easily made if you grow marigolds yourself, and it is a lovely natural beauty tonic for the bath. To make, combine cider vinegar with a handful of marigold flowers and heat till nearly boiling. Cover and steep overnight, then strain and add to your bath for a healing and skin-soothing effect. This is particularly good for very dry or chapped skin, and a few drops will take away the pain of burns. The vinegar is also useful for a baby suffering nappy rash. Be sure to dilute it, preferably by adding a tablespoon to baby's bathwater.

It is worth taking the time to pot up a supply of marigold ointment. Simple to prepare, it has a variety of uses, being ideal as a breast massage cream and for soothing nappy rash. Take 3 tablespoons of pure white lard and melt over a low heat. Add 2 tablespoons of bruised marigold petals and simmer. Cover until quite cold. Warm again, drain marigold petals and pour into a clean, clear glass jar before storing in the fridge.

In a recent example of natural health care knowledge being accepted by the medical profession, marigold oil was used successfully in clinical trials in an English hospital to treat corns and calluses. Marigold oil has long been used by natural therapists in creams and tinctures to treat athlete's foot, verrucae and other fungal infections. It can be obtained from a herbalist or a specialist health food store supplier and applied to corns with a pad over a 10- to 12-week period.

CAMPHOR

This is derived from the wood of a tree native to eastern Asia, *Cinnamomum camphora*, and is used as a natural remedy throughout the world. Spirits of camphor is the natural remedy for pimples that I like better than anything else, and I never go on a trip without taking some with me. Just pat it on the pimple every time you think of it, and if the pimple is just beginning it will dry up and disappear. If the pimple already has a head on it, apply a very hot damp cloth till the head practically pops out of its own accord, with only the gentlest squeezing. Then pat the camphor on. It will sting slightly, but it prevents infection and also makes the blotch heal rapidly.

Spirits of camphor is great for insect bites, too. It has also been used externally for healing bruises and sprains and for the pain of rheumatism. Camphor has been used therapeutically, in very small controlled doses, for whooping cough and vomiting because of its sedative and antispasmodic effects. (Note that camphor oil should not be taken internally without the supervision of a qualified natural therapist.)

Tip:
Combine a teaspoon of tincture of marigold with lanolin and apricot oil to soften and protect dry lips.

Tip:
Put a few drops of spirits of camphor or camphor oil in water used to rinse the face after cleansing. It will help to whisk away last traces of oils and fats, and any residue from soaps or creams that may block the pores.

CARAWAY

Caraway (*Carum carvi*) seeds are known to help stomach spasms and flatulence and they act as an antiseptic and stimulant to the body. Caraway is also useful for treating digestive problems in infants. For colic, try crushing some seeds and simmering them in milk or formula for 20 minutes, before straining the liquid and giving it to the child. The seeds can also be cooked and mashed, and used warm as a poultice for bruises and sprains. They are said to increase the milk supply in nursing mothers, and were once used in aphrodisiac charms, being thought to encourage fidelity between lovers. Caraway seed oil may be used to treat toothache in much the same way as clove oil, although it has a milder effect; to use, apply oil to a clean cotton ball or bud and hold gently against the affected area.

CARDAMOM

Cardamom seeds (Elettaria cardamomum) are to be found in a large reed-like plant which grows primarily throughout Sri Lanka and South-East Asia. They were first chewed by the ancient Egyptians to whiten their teeth and freshen their breath, and today are harvested and exported for use worldwide in herbal medicine, as well as for culinary use.

Cardamom seeds have strong carminative and stimulant properties, meaning they may be useful in treating digestive and circulatory conditions. An infusion of cardamom helps to prevent flatulence and colic, especially when these disorders are accompanied by sensations of cold, for cardamom has a notable 'warming' effect. A tea may be taken for indigestion and to stimulate the appetite; herbalists may prescribe cardamom as an accompaniment to laxatives or other medicines intended to treat a gastrointestinal upset.

CARROT

Carrots (Daucus carota) are commonly used for diuretic and stimulating purposes by naturopaths and nutritionists.

Carrot soup, for instance, is an effective remedy for nervous diarrhoea and is easily digestible for those suffering stomach and intestinal problems. The carrot's high potassium content also promotes a diuretic action, and if two to three raw carrots are eaten each day, this is an effective natural remedy for fluid retention. One or two cups per day of freshly processed carrot juice are very helpful in cases of stomach acidity and heartburn.

Tip:

Carrots have an unexpected bonus as a natural remedy, being an excellent aid for breakouts on the skin. Finely grate two or three medium carrots and apply pulp to any rash, pimples or acne area. Leave on for 10 minutes, then rinse off.

CASCARA

Cascara (*Rhamnus purshiana*) or cascara sagrada is possibly the world's best known laxative, being a potent stimulant. It has a gentler action than other natural remedies or herbs, and is less likely to cause griping or cramp-like pain, which can occur with harsh mineral oil-based laxatives. It is native to the mountainous areas of north-west America, and the Spanish explorers sent samples of the bark back to Spain, hailing it as a 'wonder of the New World'.

Today, cascara essence is included in a wide variety of over-the-counter products for constipation; it is also the 'magic ingredient' in many drugs prescribed by doctors for the same problem. It may also be taken as a tea — 1 to 3 g of the powdered dried bark in a cup of hot water, prior to retiring for the night, should do the trick, although it is quite bitter to the taste. It is advisable to purchase the bark rather than attempt to harvest it yourself — unlike the majority of other herbs, cascara bark should not be used for at least a year after it has been dried; otherwise it can cause intestinal cramping. By the same token, pregnant women should avoid cascara and all products containing it.

CASSIA

The bark of the evergreen tree *Cinnamomum cassia*, also known as Chinese cinnamon, has a fragrant odour which is reminiscent of cinnamon but a much stronger taste. This bark contains certain volatile oils and tannins which have a warming and soothing effect when used as a tonic and an aid to digestion. Oil of cassia (known in the USA, rather oddly, as 'oil of cinnamon') is what is known to herbalists as a carminative, meaning it is an aid to digestion; it also has antispasmodic effects. Pieces of the bark are included in potpourri mixes and the oil is sometimes used in the commercial manufacture of incense pastilles and sticks.

CASTOR OIL

Castor oil, obtained from the castor bean (*Ricinus communis*), an Indian shrub, is a very rich and emollient natural remedy for skin and hair conditions. Barbra Streisand was once quoted as rubbing castor oil on her face and neck each day. She said it was a trick employed by many actresses, as it kept the wrinkles at bay. Castor oil does indeed possess remarkable 'drawing' powers, helping to clear the skin of impurities when used cosmetically, as well as tone the internal organs when used medicinally. It is also well known as a nonirritating and highly effective purgative and laxative; it was once used to 'dose' children and rid them of worms, and as a treatment for colic and constipation. An odd old use for castor oil was, supposedly, to stimulate the milk in nursing mothers, this idea hailing from the Canary Islands.

For very delicate or weak hair, try using a drop of rosemary oil in warmed castor oil. This pale yellow thick oil is particularly strengthening. An old folk remedy for falling hair consists of alternate applications of castor oil and white iodine for 4 days. (The juice of a lemon rubbed into the scalp is also said to be good for falling hair.) Castor oil will also improve the condition of weak or overly short eyelashes and eyebrows. Apply nightly with a small brush.

Tip:

Try this as a treatment for fragile hair. Warm ½ cup of castor oil, massage it well into the scalp and comb through the hair with a wide-toothed comb. Heat a damp towel in a slow oven and wrap about the head, leaving for 30 minutes until cool. This will facilitate the absorption of the oil and is very good for split ends. Shampoo with a mild shampoo.

CATMINT

The tiny scented leaves and pretty pale pinky-mauve flowers of catmint or catnip (*Nepeta cataria*) make a delightful tea which has the effect of relaxing the nerves and muscles. Its properties were first noted by early herbalists, who observed cats rolling ecstatically around the low-growing bushes and then stretching out to sun themselves.

By association, it became a natural remedy for sleeplessness, nervous tension and stress. Catmint tea is still regarded as particularly useful for small children, having a soothing and tranquillising effect as well as helping to relieve pain and bring down a temperature by promoting perspiration, what is known as a diaphoretic effect by natural therapists. It may be used as a natural remedy for colds, upper respiratory tract infections and fevers, particularly where there is a feeling of congestion in the airways, sinuses or middle ear. Some research has pointed to catmint's use as a bowel and gastrointestinal tonic, and it has been used to relieve severe colic, nervous dyspepsia and a wide range of digestive upsets. Cooled catmint tea is a very old remedy for haemorrhoids. Catmint also has cosmetic applications, being useful as a hair rinse and as a treatment for itchy or scabby scalps.

CAYENNE

At the onset of a cold there are many herbal remedies that will help to reduce the severity of the symptoms. Cayenne (*Capsicum minimum*), the familiar red and hot spice, may be made into a tea, for instance, and will quickly and thoroughly warm a chilled body and stimulate the circulation. This is due to the action of one of its principal ingredients, an alkaloid named capsaicin, which is a strong circulatory stimulant, helping to increase the blood flow through all the body tissues and to increase the subjective feeling of heat.

Cayenne pepper, surprisingly, has a very powerful internal and external styptic action. A tiny bit of the powder can stop bleeding from a cut and a few grains taken with a large glass of water can help relieve internal bruising or bleeding. It also stimulates gastric secretions and so acts as a carminative, helping to reduce flatulence, indigestion and colic.

CEDARWOOD

Cedarwood (*Juniperus virginiana*) is the source of an oil much used in bath preparations, colognes and soap making. Cedarwood chips are used in sachets and potpourri mixes, too.

CEDARWOOD BATH OIL

1 ½ cups olive oil

4 tablespoons alcohol (or 80 proof vodka)

1 tablespoon oil of cedarwood

Combine the olive oil and cedarwood oil, add alcohol and shake well before use.

CELANDINE

The leaves and flowers of the lesser celandine or pile-wort (*Ranunculus ficaria*) are both an effective natural remedy for haemorrhoids, due to its astringent properties, and for flabby or sagging skin, which can often result from weight reduction or cellulite loss. For haemorrhoids, the leaves can be pulped and added to an ointment, or an infusion of the leaves (made by combining about 30 g of leaves in 600 ml of boiling water, and straining before use) may be drunk two to three times daily.

To prepare a stimulating treatment for flabby skin, place 30 g of the leaves in a non-aluminium saucepan with a litre of water and bring to the boil, then simmer for 8 to 10 minutes. Remove from heat and allow to cool. Strain the mixture through a nonmetallic sieve, pressing down well on the plant material to extract the essence. To use, sit in the bath and vigorously rub this liquid over the affected area in a friction manner at least once daily. This liquid may also be used as a remedy for corns or eczema.

Tip:

From a score of alleged wart cures, one of the most reliable is made from celandine. Apply the raw juice from this plant, made by pulping the leaves and the stems and sieving them to remove the fibrous matter, to the offending wart every night and morning.

CELERY

Celery (*Apium graveolens*) is a good source of potassium and sodium in the diet, but it is the essential oils contained in this plant that have a specific use as a natural remedy.

Celery seeds contain a volatile oil known as apiol, along with flavonoids, and can be used as an aperient or diuretic. The extracted juice of the plant is also an effective medicine, and may be used as a digestive tonic and uterine stimulant; both the seeds and the plant itself can be used in arthritic conditions and also to stimulate milk flow in nursing mothers. One tablespoon of celery juice two to three times a day an hour before meals, or 1 to 3 g of the dried seed three times a day, is an effective dosage for rheumatism and gout (as this increases the elimination of uric acid), as well as for tendencies towards overweight, lack of appetite and deficiency-related diseases.

A wineglassful of celery juice, sweetened with honey if desired, may be taken before meals as a digestive tonic. It should not be used to excess when acute kidney problems exist. For clearing skin problems, celery — either as a vegetable, or brewed in a tea, or taken in supplemental form — is highly recommended. Raw grated celery, combined with flaxseed, makes a useful poultice for swellings and abrasions.

Tip:
At bedtime, a glass of celery juice will induce sound sleep.

Note: Celery seed sold for horticultural use is usually treated with a fungicide; do not use these seeds internally as a natural remedy. Seek out the untreated seeds or seed-based products (such as capsules, tablets and tea), or harvest your own seeds from home-grown celery.

CHAMOMILE

Chamomile (*Matricaria chamomilla*) has long been cultivated as a medicinal herb and early documents refer to chamomile compresses as being used for healing all manner of ailments, from abscesses to rheumatism. No doubt due to its healing prowess, it was even believed to be a sacred herb. In Anglo-Saxon England, *maythen* (as it was then known) was much respected, and the very old manuscript 'Nine Herbs Charm' advises us to 'Remember . . . that he never yielded his life because of infection after Mayweed was dressed for his food'.

The tiny, daisy-like blossoms of this fragrant European

herb are rich in azulene, a blue oil that soothes skin irritations and promotes healing. Regular bathing in chamomile water was once widely touted to reduce wrinkles. This is not surprising since chamomile's mildly astringent effect does clean and tighten the pores, while its natural glycosides (plant sugars) brighten the complexion.

Chamomile flowers are most commonly used to make a soothing tea. Today chamomile is often sold both by itself and as a blended tea. Brew chamomile tea in the same way as ordinary tea; you may sweeten it with honey to taste, but don't add milk. In early times, chamomile tea was said to prevent nightmares, soothe frazzled nerves and to treat menstrual cramps and digestive upsets. Chamomile's fragrance has a definite calming effect — a steam inhalation can be used to calm sleeplessness and hysteria while a very mild tea may be given to a baby suffering from colic.

'To comfort the braine, smell to camomill . . . wash measurably, sleep reasonably; delight to hear melody and singing . . .' Ram's Little Dodoen, 1606

A soothing oil is also sold which is made from the flowers and leaves. This oil, or 'essential oil', may be variously used for speeding wound healing, treating burns and bruises, earache, neuralgia and toothache. Chamomile is also well known as an ingredient in rinses and conditioners for the hair. A bright yellow flower, chamomile seems best suited for blonde hair, but all colours benefit from the brightening effect of a chamomile rinse that cuts through dulling soap film. It is particularly effective when mixed with rosewater. The Vikings are said to have used chamomile tea to rinse their hair, thus enhancing their blondness! Chamomile tea and/or an oil

Tip:
To an infusion of chamomile tea, add juice of a lemon and enough kaolin (see Kaolin) to form a paste. Work through hair and leave for an hour before rinsing out. The process can be speeded up if you dry the paste with a hair drier or sit out in the sunshine while it's on.

Tip:
Adding a strong brew of chamomile tea to bathwater will have a soothing effect on dry or sunburned skin.

made by steeping the purchased dried flowers in a fine carrier oil, such as apricot kernel oil, may be used as a rich hair conditioner. Both are particularly useful for those suffering from dandruff or for babies with cradle cap.

CHARCOAL

A 'sour tummy' is sometimes caused by insufficient hydrochloric acid secretions, meaning the food does not break down quickly enough in the stomach. A reduced concentration of hydrochloric acid also favours the growth of the micro-organisms that produce bad breath. Sometimes charcoal tablets taken between meals can do the trick. The charcoal both absorbs the odour and the bacteria that may be causing it, giving your digestive system a chance to re-establish a balance.

CHERVIL

Chervil (Anthriscus cerefolium) has blood-cleansing properties. It is a digestive, and a tea made from the flowers and leaves may be used to increase perspiration, thus lowering the temperature of a feverish patient. The leaves are gently astringent and a light infusion may be used as a skin freshener. Pliny the Elder favoured chervil as a medicinal herb, saying it would improve the digestion and give an appetite to girls who were 'pale and wan'. He also recommended chervil tea and chervil steeped in vinegar as cures for hiccups.

Fresh chervil juice or an infusion of chervil may be used as a facial wash of particular benefit to those with blemished skin. For best results, a strong tea made from chervil should be taken at the same time, thus helping to cleanse the internal system of any impurities, too, which may be helping the skin to 'break out'.

In the 17th century, Nicolas Culpeper wrote in his *Compleat Herball* that chervil could be used 'to dissolve congealed or clotted blood in the body, or that which is clotted by bruises, falls, etc . . . the juice or distilled water thereof being drunk and the bruised leaves laid to the place'. A hot poultice made from chervil and mashed potatoes is one of those odd old country remedies for a bruise or sprain that really do work. Herbalist John Parkinson went on to say that the long taproots could also be cooked and eaten candied in a syrup 'to warme and comfort a phlegmaticke stomacke'.

CHICKWEED

Chickweed (*Stellaria media*), also known as starweed and satinflower, is a gentle healing herb; it may be used medicinally or, increasingly, as a culinary herb in salads. It is high in nutritional value, containing relatively large amounts of vitamins A and C. Chickweed is also a traditional and safe mild eye herb that can be used as a soothing lotion or on sterile compresses. It has a marked strengthening effect on tired eyes and will reduce inflammations. For this latter reason chickweed is often an ingredient in different types of anti-inflammatory creams, lotions, cosmetics or tonics which may be purchased in a health food store or pharmacy. Chickweed's soothing and demulcent effects mean that it may be used as an ingredient in tonics for treating inflammations of the lungs and indigestion, and in ointments for treating haemorrhoids, sores, eczema and chilblains. It is also beneficial in treating constipation.

To make a compress, take a handful of fresh chickweed, wash it and shake it dry, taking care to check that no grit or bugs adhere to it. Then place it in a non-aluminium saucepan with about 2 tablespoons of milk and simmer for approximately 10 minutes. Remove the mixture from the heat and crush to a pulp, pressing the herb well into the milk to make a thick texture. Allow the pulp to cool and use directly on closed eyes; alternatively, soak pieces of clean lint or cotton in the herb mixture and lay them over the eyes for 10 minutes.

CHICORY

Many spring herbs such as chicory or succory (*Chicorium intybus*) have reputations as cleansers or purifiers and are traditionally eaten at Easter or the Jewish Passover. Rather like its cousin, the dandelion, chicory is slightly bitter, which has the effect of increasing the secretion of digestive juices, stimulating a sluggish stomach, helping digestion and restoring the appetite. Chicory is often used as an ingredient in natural coffee substitutes. Try blanching chicory leaves and including them in a salad, or take an infusion of chicory 30 minutes before eating. The juice from the fresh root may be prescribed by a herbalist as a laxative and tonic. The leaves may also be pulped and used warm as a poultice for inflamed skin.

CHIVES

Although the protective and curative powers of garlic have been noted throughout the ages, surprisingly little attention has been paid to its cousin, chives (*Allium schoenoprasum*). The Chinese used chives in poultices to stem bleeding and would also bind pulped chives over bites and abscesses, believing this would act as an antidote to the poison. Nicolas Culpeper, on the other hand, wrote disparagingly of chives in his *Herball* of 1649, saying 'They send up very hurtful vapours to the braine, causing troublesome sleep'.

Although chives are not as strong a natural remedy as garlic, they still have quite marked tonic and antiseptic effects, being rich in sulphur. The diluted juice may be applied externally to sores and taken regularly as part of the diet. Chives' antiseptic action helps prevent infection and the accumulation of harmful bacteria in the colon and stomach. Most recently, research has indicated that chives are mildly antibiotic and therefore beneficial to kidney and stomach function. Remember this next time you are concocting a light savoury dish for a recuperating invalid. Similarly, chives have a reputation for stimulating the appetite.

Tip:

Not only the leaves and flowers of chives are edible and healthful. Pickle the tiny bulbs as a gourmet treat for anyone who enjoys savoury foods.

CHOLINE

Choline is a member of the B group of vitamins. It is the biochemical precursor of acetylcholine, a transmitter of nerve impulses within the body: too little, and problems such as forgetfulness and tremor can result. This nutrient is also involved in the correct metabolism of fats and reduces excessive deposits of fat and cholesterol within the circulatory system. It is especially beneficial to mental and nervous system health. Poor memory can be improved with choline. Some researchers have suggested it may help with Alzheimer's disease and heart palpitations.

The highest amount of choline is present in lecithin, usually obtained from soya beans. Other good food sources include brewer's yeast, wheat germ, egg yolk, brains, liver, green leafy vegetables, peas, nuts and fruits. Signs of a possible dietary deficiency include headaches, dizziness, tinnitus (ringing in the ears), hypoglycaemia, fatigue and muscle weakness.

CIDER VINEGAR

Small amounts of cider vinegar and water will often relieve indigestion and heartburn. If the treatment works, it frequently indicates that the body has a shortage of acids in the digestive system. Apple cider vinegar and honey (1 tablespoon of each) in a cup of warm water may also be used to rebalance the body after illness.

Tip:

Severe dandruff? Make a strong infusion of nettles and add to an equal amount of cider vinegar. Massage into scalp morning and night. Or try the following treatment. Beat 2 egg yolks into ½ cup of warm water and massage into scalp and hair. Leave for 10 minutes, then rinse out with warm water. Now massage 2 tablespoons of apple cider vinegar into the scalp and hair and leave for 2 to 3 minutes before washing out.

Soap, which is alkaline, tends to strip the natural acid mantle of the skin. Rinsing your skin with apple cider vinegar will also help to restore the correct acid:alkaline balance and relieve any itching or dryness. Add 1 cup straight to the bathwater or pat straight vinegar on the affected areas with a cotton pad or cotton wool ball. Or mix equal parts of vinegar and hot water. When cooled, use this liquid as a facial wash, patting it on with cotton wool balls. This has a tonic effect on the complexion as a whole, in addition to helping to refine the pores.

A final rinse of cider vinegar also helps to protect and condition the hair by removing residual alkaline traces after shampooing and restoring the natural acidic balance of the scalp. Cider vinegar also has an astringent effect on oily hair. Any herbs can be infused, singly or mixed, in this final vinegar rinse, leaving your hair sweet-smelling and very shiny. After shampooing, rinse your hair with lots of tepid water. Once it is entirely soap-free, pour the cider vinegar rinse through your hair, then blot it dry and gently untangle with your fingers and a wide-toothed comb.

Try any of the following additions to your cider vinegar hair rinse, depending on your hair's requirements: horsetail and sage add shine and enhance colour; parsley helps clear dandruff and restore thickness of thinning hair; rosemary darkens dark hair and imparts a lovely fragrance; chamomile and yarrow are both purported to stimulate hair growth.

CINNAMON

King Solomon was plagued with indigestion and he used cinnamon (Cinnamomum zeylanicum) to treat this complaint. I can vouch for his wisdom, having kept a jar of the dried powdered bark on the kitchen shelf throughout both my pregnancies. Steep 2 teaspoons of the powder in boiling water for 15 minutes, cool, then sip slowly 1 hour before each meal. This is a most effective natural remedy for all sorts of digestive complaints, including flatulence, diarrhoea, nausea and cramps.

Cinnamon tea is also an antispasmodic, making it useful for preventing both internal cramping, such as can accompany menstruation, or 'night cramps' of the leg, calf and foot. (Leg cramps may be further alleviated by supplementing the diet with calcium and an increased intake of vitamin B_6; also, vegetable oils will help improve circulation.) Cooled cinnamon tea or cinnamon oil, distilled from the bark and leaves of the cinnamon tree, is useful on a compress for toothache.

Try the following cooling, refreshing and mildly antiseptic preparation, either for sprinkling in the bath or for splashing over the body after bathing.

Tip:

To strengthen your nails, soak them in apple cider vinegar daily, then paint with white iodine. Drink a glassful of the vinegar three times daily — this is also good for your general health.

Tip:

The aromatic bark of the cinnamon tree may be infused in water and added to bathwater; it will be wonderfully fragrant as well as uplifting and refreshing to jaded nerves.

Tip:
A few drops of oil of cinnamon added to olive oil can be used as a soothing and warming rub.

AROMATIC CINNAMON VINEGAR

500 *ml cider vinegar*

2 *drops oil of cloves*

10 *drops oil of cinnamon*

5 *drops oil of lemon*

1 *to* 2 *drops oil of bergamot or neroli*

Mix thoroughly and shake well before use.

CINQUEFOIL

Cinquefoil (*Potentilla reptans*), or five-fingered grass, was first recorded by 17th century herbalist Nicolas Culpeper as being useful as an anti-inflammatory and cooling medicine, both externally for use on the skin and internally. The leaves may be brewed to make an infusion which has an astringent effect on the skin; this may be added to the bath, or diluted and used as a facial toner. Cinquefoil's astringent properties also mean it is a remedy for internal problems such as diarrhoea; it is an occasional ingredient in purchased syrups for sore throats.

CLEAVERS

Tonics may be necessary after illness and some individuals need them more in the spring to get a sluggish post-winter body moving, or when under work or family stress. Cleavers (*Galium aparine*) tea, also called goosegrass or hairif tea, was a traditional Anglo-Saxon spring tonic, and is commonly prescribed today by herbalists as an uplifter for patients suffering depression. It is a mild laxative and diuretic and may be used as a tonic for digestive and urinary complaints such as cystitis. It also helps to lower the body temperature and regulate the lymphatic system, making it of use in treating a feverish patient. Some new research points to its use in reducing or stopping tumour formation.

Cleavers is also a useful beauty herb. For a herbal hair and scalp lotion, prepare, fresh each week, an infusion using cleavers. Massage the scalp with this daily. For dry, brittle hair, add essential oil of cleavers to the mixture for extra benefit. Where dandruff is present, a pinch of nettle will help dispose of the problem.

CLOVES

Cloves, the dried unopened flower buds of Eugenia aromatica, were once burned to scent and disinfect rooms. This custom was recorded before the birth of Christ, when it was a favourite incense in the Chinese Han Court. In addition to their spicy fragrance, cloves provided a therapeutic benefit, having strong antibacterial properties. Through ancient and mediaeval times, cloves were imported from the Middle East to Europe and used to pickle and preserve meats. In the 17th century, sponges soaked in clove-scented oil were held beneath the noses of victims of the plague. Doctors tending the victims attempted to keep the disease at bay by breathing through an odd type of mask that had a 'beak' filled with cloves.

Tip:
Add a few drops of clove oil to a tepid footbath for aching feet.

Cloves are stimulating, aromatic and the most carminative of all the aromatic spices. They are an excellent natural remedy to reduce griping action of purgatives. They are often added to herb teas to settle an upset stomach and vomiting. Clove oil will stop the pain of a toothache if a few drops are placed on cotton wool and held against the tooth in question. Clove oil is also used commercially in toothpastes, mouthwashes, and in ointments and rubs for rheumatism and arthritis for its warming, stimulating and locally anaesthetic effects. A few drops of the oil in water will stop vomiting and clove tea may be taken for nausea.

COCOA BUTTER

A thick, creamy oil used as an emollient to lubricate the skin, cocoa butter (*Theobroma cacao*) is a very common ingredient in natural cosmetics and creams. You can also buy the pure cocoa butter, and use this either by itself or to prepare homemade natural remedies.

For hands, cocoa butter is an effective softener. Use just as is, or combine equal parts of almond oil, cocoa butter and white wax (preferably beeswax). Melt together in a double boiler and stir until cool. Keep in a dark glass jar, labelled.

Cocoa Butter Neck Smoother

1 *tablespoon cocoa butter*

1 *tablespoon lanolin*

½ *cup wheat germ oil*

Combine all ingredients in a non-aluminium saucepan and heat over a low flame till melted together. Adding 1 or 2 teaspoons of purified water may help to make the mixture more spreadable. Remove from heat, pour into a clean glass jar and cap securely. Store in the refrigerator, shaking well before use. To use, apply to the neck using long, smooth, upwards-and-outwards strokes.

COCONUT OIL

Coconut oil is an inexpensive and effective natural remedy and cosmetic which should be present in every home medicine chest. It is a white semisolid saturated fat, which forms the basis of nearly all cosmetics, soaps, shampoos and skin and hair preparations which are commercially available. It is an excellent lubricant for all dry skin conditions, either for use by itself or as a base for preparing herb oils. In particular, coconut oil has a long history of use in those areas where the tree is native, namely Malaysia and tropical Asia.

A liquefied detergent base is prepared from coconut oil, and this is the surfactant used in most natural brands of shampoos, foam cleansers or bath preparations as it is biodegradable and free from additives, dyes and perfumes.

COD LIVER OIL

In addition to being taken internally as a liquid supplement of vitamin A, vitamin D and certain essential fatty acids, either neat or via capsules for those who do not like the taste, a little known (and inexpensive) use for cod liver oil is for nappy rash. I used it on my babies, and it was so wonderfully healing that I now recommend it for all manner of other skin problems. It works like a charm on blotches, rashes, pimples, cold sore blisters, or what have you. It is probably only a matter of time before an entrepreneurial natural foods company includes cod liver oil in its commercially available skin cosmetic ranges, but to the best of my knowledge, at present it is listed as an ingredient in only a few ointments.

COLTSFOOT

An infusion made from the leaves of coltsfoot (*Tussilago farfara*), also known as the aptly named cough wood, is very soothing and may help certain chest complaints such as bronchitis, persistent coughing or breathlessness. It is an expectorant, meaning it loosens mucus, and it also has demulcent properties, meaning it will soothe any irritation in the lungs or digestive system. Externally, it may be made up in a lotion to prevent thread veins on the face. Coltsfoot was first listed in Culpeper's 17th century herbal as being an anti-inflammatory herb for the skin and skin eruptions, and also an internal preparation. It is particularly useful for those with dry skin which feels stretched and tight, becomes easily chapped in cold weather, flaky in hot sun and is prone to wrinkles. Coltsfoot is sometimes listed as an ingredient in rich moisturising creams and lotions, for it is an emollient as well as an astringent. The leaves may be pulped and used warm as a poultice for sores, skin inflammations or infected insect bites.

Tip:

Coltsfoot is beneficial for a flushed complexion and dilated veins: make up as a weak tea and use as a skin lotion on a compress. To make, add 1 teaspoon of crumbled dried leaves to 150 ml boiling water, infuse for 10 minutes, then strain.

COMFREY

Comfrey (*Symphytum officinale*), also known as knit-bone and boneset, has been used for centuries to heal bruises and other irritations of the skin. Swellings of all sorts calm down when washed with comfrey tea or an infusion of comfrey. It is lovely as a footbath for swollen or infected feet. To make the bath, combine a handful of chopped peeled comfrey root with a litre of boiling water. Steep, then chill. You can also dress a wound on the foot by soaking the dressing with a strong infusion of comfrey.

Folk healers have long used comfrey to heal all sorts of sports injuries, including damaged cartilage. Recent research has shown that this healing ability is due to the presence of allantoin and choline, which stimulate the circulation and help red blood cells to reproduce, thus speeding healing. Apply either the mashed green leaves or gummy boiled roots directly to the area, or encase in a cotton cloth and bind on tightly. A poultice of mashed comfrey will also reduce swelling and heal skin tears and cuts. Fresh poultices of comfrey leaves will heal almost any body sore, including chapped nipples. In many parts of Europe, nurses once applied the hollow part of the comfrey plant root directly over the sore nipple of a new mother. Comfrey will help heal many mouth abrasions. After tooth extraction, put a few drops of boiling water on a little pad which contains a teaspoon of chopped dried comfrey root and hold over the place to reduce inflammation and swelling. Herbalists may prescribe comfrey for internal use to treat ulcers or bronchitic conditions.

Tip:

Make the following comfrey root lotion, which suits any skin type. However, its toning and soothing properties make it especially suitable for those with particularly dry or sensitive skins. Peel a piece of comfrey root about 10 cm long, place in a non-aluminium saucepan with 150 ml water and bring to the boil. Strain and allow the lotion to cool. It may be bottled and stored in the refrigerator for up to 4 weeks.

CORIANDER

Coriander (*Coriandrum sativum*) has long been used as a culinary herb; it is also a traditional digestive aid. It was much used in early Greek medicine, and Roman physicians are thought to have popularised coriander amongst the Egyptians, both as a medicine and as a food preservative. Early monks grew coriander in their monastery gardens or 'physicke gardens', and prescribed an infusion of the seeds for flatulence, nausea and indigestion. Most commonly, they were used as a flavouring agent to disguise sour-tasting herbal mixtures. In fact, coriander is still often used as an ingredient in commercial cough syrups for this reason, as well as being an active ingredient in all manner of digestive compounds and tonics to stimulate the appetite and to relieve colic and flatulence.

Small quantities of coriander oil are sometimes used in natural cosmetics, mainly to enhance fragrances in creams, lotions and perfumes. Probably the best known product which today features coriander is Eau de Cologne. This light and popular perfume is a descendant of the famous 17th century Carmelite water, developed by French Carmelite monks as a preparation for cleansing and purifying the skin. In Middle Eastern countries, coriander seeds were pounded with goat's milk to make a paste which was supposed to soften and bleach the skin.

The leaves have been used until quite recently in ointments to help soothe joint pains and skin irritations. This is a very old use, in fact, dating back to 1551 when William Turner wrote that 'Coriandre layd to wythe breade and barly mele is good for Saint Antoynes fyre [erysipelas, a skin disorder]'. A weak infusion or tea of coriander may be given to children suffering from colic and also to older people who may find that food 'repeats' on them unpleasantly. Mix a handful of pounded seeds with a teaspoon of honey and steep in a cup of boiling water for 5 minutes or so. Sip before and after meals.

CORNFLOUR

Many foot problems are caused by badly fitting shoes or inadequate foot care. Blisters, in particular, are due to heat friction on pressure points such as the heels, the instep and on the outer side of the soles. Protect blisters with an adhesive padding before they burst and until they have healed. Cornflour dusted over blisters soothes and helps the healing process. Cornflour is also a valuable natural remedy for relieving the sting and discomfort of sunburn.

BASIC TALC

1 cup cornflour

½ cup rice flour

½ teaspoon to 1 teaspoon essential oil of your choice

(rose, jasmine or clove, for instance)

Combine the flours, stir in the oil and store in a tightly lidded container with holes punched in the top, shaking well before each use.

CORNFLOWER

Cornflower is the common name of a lovely blue-flow-ered herb (*Centaurea cyanus*), which is also sometimes known as bluebottle and is easily grown in even the smallest of gardens. The flowers have quite remarkable properties as a natural remedy, both as a nerve-soothing tea and as a general stimulant and tonic which is helpful for dyspepsia, or to be applied externally to take the sting and itch out of insect bites. Cornflower tea also has a long traditional use as a bath for inflamed or infected eyes; many centuries ago, the French produced a famous medicinal eyewash based on cornflowers, known as Eau de Casselunette. Cornflower essence may be listed as an ingredient in some brands of eye gel or cosmetic eye balm.

CORN SILK

Diuretics stimulate the kidneys to eliminate water and are popular drugs for high blood pressure and oedema. However, they can lead to potassium deficiencies. The good news is that there are natural diuretics that work just as well for water watchers.

Many herbs are diuretics and make a pleasant tea, such as nettle and ginseng. Corn (*Zea mays*) silk, being the protective 'silk' or covering around the corncobs and inside the leaves, is another such herb. Corn silk tablets or capsules are an effective natural diuretic. This means it is a useful slimmer's aid, doubling or even quadrupling the flow of urine. It is also a useful natural remedy for most urinary problems, including cystitis, as it has a soothing and demulcent effect on the urinary tract and helps to clear toxins and cleanse internal tissues. To make a tea, infuse about 25 g dried corn silk in 500 ml boiling water for 10 to 15 minutes, strain, and drink as often as you like between meals (up to a litre a day). Corn silk tea and inhalations may also be of use in treating certain respiratory complaints, notably an irritating 'dry' cough.

COUCH GRASS

A herbal tea made from equal parts of couch grass or twitch grass (*Agropyron repens*) and peppermint has diuretic and slimming properties. Couch grass is a very old remedy for kidney and bladder difficulties, such as cystitis, and for nausea and stomach complaints. Interestingly, cats and dogs eat couch grass when they are sick.

COWSLIP

Tip:

Cowslips may be used to make a mild yet effective skin freshener. Simply simmer 1 tablespoon of the dried flowers in enough water to cover for 5 minutes, strain and bottle.

The pretty wild cowslip (*Primula veris*) is beloved by poets as a symbol of springtime and renewal the world over. The pink-edged yellow flowers are softly fragrant and very pretty. They are also a potent natural sedative and cosmetic. Seventeenth century herbalist and apothecary John Parkinson wrote that 'cowslippe flowers were good to take away spottes' and they may still be used as a beauty restorative to counter wrinkles and freckles. The petals may be brewed into a nerve-soothing tea and used to treat dizziness, nervousness, headaches, cramps and insomnia. A diluted infusion may be used externally to bathe reddened or inflamed skin conditions and to fade skin blemishes or freckles. Cowslip infusion is especially helpful for dry skin, and may be mixed in with your own usual lotion or cream for its effect. Herbalists may prescribe cowslip tea for patients with chronic bronchitis.

CRANBERRY

No doubt it was the Native Americans' use of cranberries (*Vaccinium macrocarpon*) that inspired the special cranberry sauce which accompanied the festive roast turkeys at those first Thanksgivings during the early years of American settlement. The Native Americans also showed the European settlers how they used cranberries to help heal arrow wounds and as a dye for cloth.

Cranberries contain a generous amount of vitamins C and A, plus iron, potassium and phosphorus. Due to their high vitamin C content, cranberries were used as a preventive of scurvy, being easy to store through winter and on long sea voyages. This high vitamin C content also helps to explain why cranberries, mixed to a paste with buttermilk, were once used as a bleach for freckles and as a general skin tonic. The berries do have an astringent and lightening effect when used on the skin as a natural cosmetic.

Tip:
One way to lessen or lighten freckles — though they can rarely be removed — is to crush fresh cranberries and rub the pulp into the skin.

Most intriguing is recent research which points to cranberries being useful as a natural remedy for cystitis. It seems that eating the berries regularly, or taking the pure juice as a supplement, has the effect of countering recurrent bouts of this infection. The juice helps to acidify the urine and thus clear any mild infection and relieve the symptoms of itching.

CRANESBILL

Cranesbill (*Geranium maculatum*), the geranium of the Middle Ages, was first listed in Mayster Jon Gardener's *The Feate of Gardenynge*, the earliest known treatise on growing and using herbs. The formal name was derived from the Greek *geranos*, meaning crane, a reference to the plant's branched carpels. The leaves have a high tannin content and were used as an astringent tonic and gargle. The root also has strong astringent properties, and may be pulped and applied, warm, to sores, wounds, swellings and bruises of all kinds. Cranesbill is a natural remedy for diarrhoea; it can be made into a tincture or a strong decoction and applied to mouth ulcers or haemorrhoids. It is sometimes used as an ingredient in natural deodorants for its astringent and mildly antiperspirant effects.

CUCUMBER

Cucumber's (*Cucumis sativus*) ability to eliminate water from the body makes it very important for those with heart and kidney problems. It also helps dissolve uric acid accumulations such as kidney and bladder stones. The seeds were once used to expel worms from the body. Constipation is helped greatly by cucumber salad. The best cucumbers to use are those fully ripe, when starting to turn yellow.

For skin and cosmetic uses, cucumber juice can be applied to the skin as a toning, refreshing lotion, or blended into a cream; it is excellent as an inclusion in any ointment or lotion used for treating burns, chafing, or dry or flaking skin. To make cucumber juice, wash the cucumbers thoroughly and then cut them, with the skin on, into small pieces. Put in an earthenware or porcelain dish, pour enough hot water over them to cover, put over a low heat and let simmer for half an hour or more. Be careful not to burn them. Then strain the mixture through a colander. Another way is to cut the cucumbers into very small pieces and mash them to a pulp. Then squeeze through cheesecloth or a sieve. This method gives you the pure fresh juice, or essence of cucumber. (A blender is useful here.)

Cucumber juice is an old favourite from way back and appears in many beauty care recipes and first aid tips, one of the best of which is this cleansing tonic, which is also very helpful in treating chapped hands.

Cucumber Cleanser

90 ml cucumber juice

90 ml distilled witch hazel

45 ml rosewater

Combine all ingredients in a lidded jar and shake well to mix. Rub into the skin thoroughly, and then rinse off with tepid water.

Another useful cucumber cleanser can be easily made. Peel half a cucumber and blend it in the food processor until you have a smooth liquid, then put this through a sieve. Combine with 250 ml whole milk and blend well. This will keep well in the refrigerator for up to 3 days.

DAMIANA

Aphrodisiacs have been sought by every culture through history. The early explorers of the New World in the 16th century noted the Native Americans' use of damiana (*Turnera diffusa*) and commenced a booming trade in its export to Europe as a tonic and aphrodisiac. The leaves and stems of damiana seem to act as a tonic to the sexual system when taken as a tea. It is also a common ingredient in various 'women's tonics' and antidepressant formulas, having a beneficial tonic effect on the female organs.

DANDELION

Tip:

Apply the white juice from a dandelion stem daily to get rid of warts.

The root of one of my favourite wildflowers, the dandelion (*Taraxacum officinale*), is available as a coffee substitute in health food stores. It is thought to be a liver cleanser and also has a tonic effect on the pancreas, spleen and female organs. It stimulates the appetite and aids digestion, too. The Arabs were among the first to identify the dandelion's medicinal prowess, and there are several references in early texts to its use as a liver tonic, and cleansing wash for the skin where sores are present.

In France, the dandelion became known colloquially as 'piss-in-bed', a direct reference to its diuretic properties. Herbalists will usually prescribe dandelion tea or a salad made with young dandelion leaves for all diseases of the liver, kidneys, gall bladder and urinary tract; in particular, dandelion tea is useful for gallstones, rheumatism, gout and fluid retention. Should you suffer from tender or engorged breasts during pregnancy, heat and mash the whole plant in a little oil before using it as a poultice to reduce pain and swelling.

Tip:

The leaves and root of the dandelion can be infused to make a lotion to revive the skin. It will have a stimulating and mildly astringent effect.

DEODORANTS

In olden days, people used herbal vinegars as natural deodorants. Depending on the herb they used, they provided a subtle perfume and also some antibacterial qualities. Herbs suitable for making such deodorant vinegars are spearmint, eau-de-Cologne mint, tea tree, marigold, thyme, yarrow or any other pungent herb which appeals.

However, not everyone has the time or inclination to brew up their own herbal vinegar. Several natural formulas found in your local health food store or pharmacy fit this description quite well. Look for those containing tea tree oil, one of nature's most effective germicides. Products containing extracts of Alpine lichen, calendula and arnica will also work to inhibit the growth of odour-forming bacteria. Soft refreshing essential oils, such as ylang-ylang, lemon and geranium, will add a light fragrance to your formula.

As a bonus, you avoid the aluminium compounds present in commercially available products, which have been accused of contributing to cancer and certain types of paralysis of the sympathetic nervous system. In particular, it is believed that people who suffer from Alzheimer's disease are not as capable of ridding their body of aluminium as others.

DILL

Dill (*Anethum graveolens*) is a popular medicinal and culinary herb. The ancient Romans chewed dill seeds to promote digestion after their lavish banquets. The seeds were chewed as a breath freshener, dill oil was added to soap and dill water was used for soothing colicky babies. Dill often appears in old herbals as a cure for

Tip:

Adding dill seeds to cooking water for cabbage or sauerkraut will help mask the odour of the cabbage and will also help to improve its digestibility.

'hicket' or 'hickocke' — hiccups. Seventeenth century herbalist Nicolas Culpeper succinctly described dill's benefits as helping 'to stayeth the belly . . and is a gallant expeller of wind'. In the New World, early American settlers came to refer to dill as 'meeting house seeds', a reference to the fact that they were chewed during long sermons to stop the parishioners' stomachs from rumbling.

Tip:

Along with basil and lavender, dill is a natural insecticide. Help keep flies and mosquitoes at bay in bug-prone parts of the house and garden with an incense burner containing 1 tablespoon of dill oil, or simply plant dill near doors and windows.

The Chinese are thought to have been the first to recommend dill water as a digestive aid for children. Dill is still an ingredient in commercially prepared 'gripe waters' for the relief of wind in babies. Make dill water yourself easily at home by steeping 1 teaspoon of bruised seeds in a teapot with 2 cups of hot water. Strain the mixture, cool and give to baby by the teaspoon before and after feeds.

Dill water may, of course, also be used to get rid of wind in adults. By association, herbalists have also prescribed dill as a natural remedy for insomnia, stomach upsets, diarrhoea, and urinary tract infections. Contemporary herbalists are likely to prescribe dill tea for pregnant women experiencing nausea. And after the baby is born, dill tea may be used to stimulate the new mother's milk production.

Interesting new research indicates that oil from dill seeds may actually inhibit the growth of certain bacteria that attach to the intestinal tract and thus may help control recurrent bouts of infectious diarrhoea. Dill seeds and dill water may also be used to sweeten bad breath. Dill is rich in minerals, especially potassium and sulphur, making it a useful tonic for the skin, hair and nails.

ECHINACEA

Echinacea or the purple coneflower (Echinacea purpurea and E. angustifolium) somewhat resembles the common black-eyed Susan of our gardens, its purple petals radiating from a dark cone-shaped centre. It is a perennial herb, and first became known to American herbalists as an effective natural remedy for all sorts of infections, fevers and bites. It has potent blood-purifying properties and is a natural antitoxin; few other plants are so beneficial as natural immune system boosters and for reducing fever. Echinacea is available in tablet and capsule form, or it may be prepared as a tea or decoction and taken internally as a botanical antibiotic to treat colds and flu, blood poisoning, boils, acne, abscessed teeth, bladder infections, tonsillitis, vaginitis and all respiratory infections.

Many herbalists now recommend that a preventive dose of echinacea be taken daily to enhance the immune system and protect against infection. Recent research in Germany saw a trial of 203 women who suffered from recurrent cystitis treated with either an anti-yeast cream or the cream in conjunction with an oral dose of echinacea. After 6 months, 60 per cent of those women treated with just the cream had had another bout of cystitis; only 16 per cent of those who had also had the echinacea tablets did.

ELDERBERRY

Grey hair can be effectively coloured with a rinse made from elderberries (Sambucus nigra). These were first used by the Romans to impart a bluish hue. You can buy elderberries pre-dried, make up an infusion and add a pinch each of salt and alum (from the chemist) for extra brightness.

ELDER FLOWERS

An infusion of elder (*Sambucus nigra*) flowers will help cure a throat infection and a hot drink of elder flower tea is one of the best traditional remedies for soothing an inflamed throat and quieting a cough. Add a pinch of powdered ginger, a few cloves and some blackcurrant syrup, to taste, and simmer to produce your own personal warming and antiseptic cough remedy. The young leaves may be brewed into a tea which is an effective diuretic, and may be used for treating urinary problems, fluid retention and rheumatism.

Elder flowers have also been used for centuries in cosmetic creams and beauty preparations, most often as a skin toner, bath additive or eyewash. They contain a semivolatile oil which is mildly astringent and a gentle stimulant to the skin. Elder flower water has long been used to clear the complexion of freckles and sunburn and to keep it in good condition. Traditionally it softens and whitens the skin. It is particularly useful in normalising excessively oily skin. The leaves may also be made into an ointment for bruises and sprains.

Tip:

Try this toner for large pores. Combine 3 tablespoons of cucumber juice with 125 ml elder flower water in a clear, clean glass bottle, then add 2 tablespoons of rosewater. Cap securely and shake well. Then, slowly, add 1 tablespoon tincture of benzoin (friar's balsam, from the chemist); shake before use. Add a little more elder flower water if the mixture is too thick for your liking.

ESSENTIAL OILS

Essential oils have long been thought to benefit the health of the mind and body. What you see for sale in your health food store or pharmacy as 'essential oils' are, in fact, the concentrated pure plant extracts of herbs and flowers long respected for both their fragrance and therapeutic value. The use of such oils, in massage, bathing or via inhalation, is known as aromatherapy. Be sure to buy your oils from a reliable and informed supplier who can advise you as to the oil's special uses. Different oils can be detoxifying, relaxing or reviving, depending on which one you choose. They are wonderful in a bath just before bed at night, or combined with a light vegetable 'carrier' oil, such as apricot kernel or almond oil, and used in massage therapy. Essential oils may also be used in the shower, on compresses to ease muscular aches, sprains and bruises, as an inhalant, as room fresheners or in beauty preparations.

Use this as a final rinse after shampooing. It will envelop you in a soft cloud of fragrance, with the added bonus of helping to offset any scalp dryness or flyaway hair after shampooing.

AROMATIC HAIR RINSE

1 *tablespoon clary sage oil*

250 ml cider vinegar

50 ml whisky

Combine all ingredients in a lidded jar. Shake well before each use, storing in the refrigerator when not in use.

EUCALYPTUS

Eucalypts are the among the most aromatic plants in the world and the volatile oil, known as eucalyptol, given off by the leaves has powerful healing, disinfectant and antiseptic properties, particularly when used as a douche or gargle. The fragrance of eucalyptus oil is head clearing, sharp and immensely refreshing. It is useful for all cold conditions related to the respiratory tract, such as coughs, asthma and bronchitis, and may be taken in inhalations, where 6 to 12 drops

Tip:

If a cold is well established, try breathing the vapour from a steaming herbal inhalant containing a few eucalyptus leaves to clear the head and soothe the respiratory tract. Sprinkle a little eucalyptus oil on the patient's pillow or handkerchief, too.

are put in a bowl of boiling water for steaming. Externally it can aid skin problems such as irritation or itching, dry cracked skin and wounds. A massage oil with a few drops of eucalyptus oil added will relieve joints afflicted with gout or rheumatism. It is also a well-known ingredient in lozenges for sore throats and coughs.

Tip:

Add a few drops of eucalyptus oil to a bath — it is wonderfully warming and stimulating and will fill the bathroom with a superb fragrance; it will also disinfect any cuts or sores and get rid of offensive body odours.

Eucalyptus globulus was dubbed 'the fever tree' because it grew in unhealthy swampy areas. Baron Ferdinand von Mueller, the controversial Director of the Botanical Gardens in Melbourne, was the first to suggest that eucalyptus oil had medicinal qualities. He sent seeds to Algiers where it was found that not only did the trees exude this refreshing and antiseptic oil, but the trees' roots helped to dry out waterlogged soil in marshy, unhealthy districts. In Sicily, eucalyptus trees were planted as a malaria preventive. The medicinal qualities of eucalyptus oil were given the official seal of approval in the 1885 edition of the British *Pharmacopoeia*.

EVENING PRIMROSE OIL

The seeds of the yellow-flowered evening primrose plant (*Oenothera biennis*), also known as the tree primrose, produce an oil which contains a high amount of gamma Linolenic acid (GLA), which has been shown to be of benefit in reducing symptoms of arthritis, skin problems and premenstrual syndrome, as well as for all kinds of inflammatory problems and immune system dysfunction. Some new research is even indicating that evening primrose oil may have promise as a treatment for multiple sclerosis. Used in conjunction with vitamin E and betacarotene (natural vitamin A), evening primrose oil has also been used to treat skin disorders, rashes, breast pain, menstrual disorders, gastrointestinal upsets and water, yet it is the oldest known skin care treatment and some allergies. The leaves and bark also contain GLA, though in lesser quantities. In traditional herbal medicine, the leaves and bark are pulped to form a gummy poultice which has a strong 'drawing' and astringent effect for wounds and skin disorders.

Tip:
Strong nails are encouraged internally by taking evening primrose oil.

EXFOLIATION

Exfoliation goes in and out of fashion as fast as soap and water, yet it is the oldest known skin care treatment and is one of the most effective. Exfoliation was mentioned in one of the oldest Egyptian papyrus rolls ever found, which dated from 1500 BC. It appears that human milk, bran and alabaster were the fashionable ingredients of the day. Other favourites that have stood the test of time include oatmeal scrubs, pumice stones, loofahs, salt and tropical fruit.

The Australian climate is a harsh one, which burns the skin, destroys collagen (the elastic fibres that keep your skin soft and youthful) and thickens the outer layer of already rough, dead cells. A sure-fire natural recipe to remove dead cells is to blend 1 cup of sea salt with 3 tablespoons of wheat germ oil. Gently massage this mixture over rough surface skin. While dead skin cells are eased away, essential oils will be added to bring a glow to lacklustre complexions.

Tip:
Cornmeal as a skin care aid is almost unheard of in Australia, but it is used extensively in America as a skin and scalp cleanser. Moisten a handful of fine meal and rub into all parts of the face and throat.

Keep a pumice stone in the bath or shower and rub it regularly over callused feet, elbows and knees to keep them soft and smooth. Dry, rough feet can be revitalised by rubbing a tablespoon of mayonnaise into each foot before bedtime. Cover with light cotton socks and rinse off any excess in the morning. Repeat for 1 week and you will notice a definite improvement in the way your feet look and feel.

EYEBRIGHT

Aching, tired eyes are a penalty of our modern life of television sets, video screens and fine print. Dark circles, puffiness and bags under the eyes can all be relieved by using eyebright (*Euphrasia officinalis*) lotion or eyebright drops or tonic (eyebright in German means 'consolation of the eyes').

Eyebright contains a plant glycoside which has a marked ability to soothe the cornea. It has anti-inflammatory and healing properties, and may be used in a compress or as a soothing eyebath; it is particularly useful for conjunctivitis in children, being mild and cooling. A combination tea of any of these herbs — elder flower, eyebright, chamomile, fennel or parsley — can be splashed onto tired eyelids for prompt relief. It can also be drunk as a general tonic.

FENNEL

There are many legends and beliefs surrounding fennel (*Foeniculum vulgare*). At one time, Greek athletes training for their Olympic games ate fennel to give them strength and to keep their weight under control. Fennel was thought to be a natural slimming agent, and a possible derivation for its Greek nickname, *marathon*, is *marathron*, meaning 'to grow thinner'. It was also thought to have special magical prowess to combat blindness. Pliny the Elder is responsible for this belief. He included fennel in many of his remedies, having first noted that when snakes rubbed against the plant after shedding their skin, their eyesight was cleared of scales. As a result, fennel began a long history as an 'eye herb', with distilled fennel water being used to treat most human eye problems.

Fennel seeds were once used to allay hunger pangs, in much the same way as dill seeds were. They were used by poor people who chewed them to stave off a rumbling tummy. Eventually, when fennel was introduced to America by the Puritans, it was said to have been favoured by church elders as a breath freshener, after they had fortified themselves for a long sermon with a shot or two of whisky. It is, of course, well known as a culinary herb, primarily because of this effect in aiding digestion. This has been known since very early times, with 17th century herbalist Nicolas Culpeper writing that 'Fennel consumes the phlegmatic humour which fish . . . annoys the body with'. Both the seeds and the fresh sprigs of the herb still make an ideal accompaniment to any oily fish recipe.

> **Tip:**
> Fennel seeds and fennel seed oil are widely employed in the confectionery trade. Take a hint, then, and use the seeds for flavouring milk-based puddings and blancmanges, and try the oil to flavour cordials, liqueurs and other homemade beverages.

Fennel is a carminative and digestive herb and has been widely used for many centuries to alleviate colic and flatulence. The seeds may either be chewed, as described above, or you can make a tea by infusing 1 to 2 teaspoons of the bruised seeds in 1 cup of boiling water. Steep for 10 minutes and drink the mixture up to three times a day. Infusions of fennel have also been used as an eyewash for tired and inflamed eyes — not just as a result of its folkloric claims described here, but because it really does have a cooling and 'clarifying' effect on the eyes. Use the same method as above, allowing the mixture to cool, of course, then either bathe the eyes with the liquid or dip squares of clean lint into it and lie down, placing the lukewarm pads over the eyes for 15 minutes.

Tip:
If anxiety is associated with stomach troubles, then chewing fennel seeds will help to calm an upset tummy.

Traditionally, fennel was said to increase the milk flow in nursing mothers and contemporary herbalists will still prescribe it for this purpose. African physicians recommend fennel for diarrhoea and indigestion. In China fennel was used as an antidote for snakebites and Nicolas Culpeper gave fennel a terrific rap when he said it would 'break wind, increase milk, cleanse the eyes from mists that hinder sight, and take away the loathings that often happen to the stomachs of sick persons'. Truly, fennel appears a versatile healing herb and natural remedy.

FENUGREEK

In North Africa and the Middle East, the seeds of the hardy annual fenugreek (*Trigonella foenum-graecum*) are commonly taken to stimulate breast milk production in nursing mothers, and are also thought to encourage 'an alluring roundness of the breast' in women generally. In India, these spicy seeds are often used for these purposes, too, as well as being a traditional condiment for curries. Perhaps this is due somehow to the seeds' active ingredient, diosgenin, which is a hormone sometimes used in oral contraceptives. They may also be made into a paste which may be applied to boils, mouth ulcers and other minor wounds.

A tea made from fenugreek will soothe a fever and help to tone up the internal organs. Sweeten with honey, to taste. This tea may also be used as a digestive aid to help with the consumption of fatty foods, and as a support treatment for acne, helping to clear minor infections and body imbalances which may be causing the skin to break out.

FEVERFEW

Anyone suffering from migraine needs professional advice, but many people find some degree of relief by chewing a leaf of fresh feverfew or pyrethrum (*Chrysanthemum parthenium*) daily. A tea of feverfew (2 teaspoons of the dried herb or 1 of the fresh to 200 ml of boiling water) is also good. Alternatively, many feverfew-based preparations, usually available in capsule or tablet form, may be purchased at your health food store or pharmacy. Feverfew is also recommended as a natural remedy for a variety of nervous disorders such as headaches and colds, fever, insomnia and hysteria. Some herbalists have used feverfew during a patient's labour to regulate contractions; however, this has varying effects and should not be attempted without medical supervision. A tincture or ointment made from feverfew has a mild antihistamine effect and is a useful natural remedy for insect bites, hives and skin rashes.

FLAX

This blue-flowered plant (*Linum usitatissimum*) is well known and respected as a natural remedy, as well as being a source of fabrics. The seeds produced by this plant may be processed to form a highly emollient oil, and this is often listed as the base of natural cosmetics. It is soothing and healing in its own right, but most importantly, it is a powerful mucilage, meaning it makes a thick and smooth-to-apply gel. This gel is an excellent first aid treatment for all manner of bruises, sprains, swellings, inflammations and burns. It is also an excellent topical treatment to reduce the itching and burning of haemorrhoids. Flaxseed gel may be used as a base or 'carrier' for other herbs or oils, too; for instance, add 1 teaspoon of mustard powder to ¾ cup of flaxseed gel and mix well to form a chest plaster for a patient with bronchitis. To make flaxseed gel, simmer 1 cup of seed with 3 cups of water until thickened. Strain the mixture through a nonmetallic sieve and thin with distilled water as required.

Tip:

It is not advisable to use any drying treatment on skin that is either naturally dry or ageing. Use fatty substances such as egg yolk as a spreader and incorporate flaxseed oil, mixing to form a sticky paste. Used as a face mask, this blend will help to revitalise skin by stimulating the pores to secrete more natural oils.

Many athletes and dancers are afflicted with lower back pain, which can be the result of direct injury, inherent weakness or simple abuse. An overall improvement in the person's nutritional status can certainly help — ensure the diet supplies adequate amounts of protein, calcium, magnesium and vitamin C, for a start. Chronic pain also responds well to hot flaxseed poultices. To make a flaxseed poultice, soak 1 cup of flaxseeds in cold water and leave overnight. Bring the mixture to the boil the next day and cook till thickened. Apply to the painful area as hot as is tolerable. This poultice is also effective on boils or other sores, as it has a strong drawing, soothing and healing action. Flaxseed oil, available from the health food store or pharmacy, can be helpful as a massage oil for chronic pain, or to ease chest pain caused by bronchitis.

Flaxseeds may also be taken as an effective bulking laxative.

FULLER'S EARTH

This is a fine, clay-like substance which is very rich in minerals and toning salts. It is used often in natural cosmetics, both for its binding properties and for its astringent and stimulating effect on the skin. It is especially useful in face masks and cleansing preparations for troubled skin. You may buy it from the pharmacy as a fine greyish powder.

Tip:

Flaxseed oil is used in a variety of soaps and creams to soothe the skin. Rub this solution into the skin while bathing, to relieve aching muscles. Combine ¼ cup flaxseed oil with ¼ cup of water and 2 tablespoons of witch hazel in a bottle or jar; cap securely and shake thoroughly before massaging into sore muscles.

GARLIC

If there is one plant that has become almost synonymous with good health, it is garlic (*Allium sativum*). The great Roman physician Galen bestowed the name 'theriaca rusticorium' upon this pungent herb. It means 'the poor man's cure-all'. Garlic was first used centuries before the birth of Jesus Christ. Today its therapeutic properties are recognised as a proven treatment for the temporary relief of colds and the symptoms of flu.

To really get back to basics, you can mash 2 cloves of garlic with 1 teaspoon of honey and take for 3 or 4 nights in succession. Many people with sinus trouble and hay fever have been helped by taking garlic regularly in this way. Many people eat raw garlic regularly as a general tonic and for its antibacterial qualities, which make it an excellent preventive medicine to guard against colds and flu, catarrh, bronchitis and persistent coughs. It is also considered beneficial in guarding against digestive problems, high blood pressure and hardening of the arteries, as well as more risky diseases such as typhoid. Or you might prefer to take a supplement, which you will find in your local health food store or pharmacy.

Garlic is rich in vitamins A, B and C, along with sulphur, iron and manganese. Its effectiveness is said to be due to the presence of the odoriferous principle, allicin. Allicin is actually created only after the garlic bulb has been crushed. Importantly, the allicin, which is responsible for garlic's antimicrobial properties, is also responsible for its odour. But allicin is all too often weakened by overprocessing. So in an attempt to reduce the odour of garlic, some preparations also manage to reduce its efficacy. Your best tip is to obtain a supplement as close as possible to the fresh garlic clove, such as one where freeze-drying technology is used. This process removes only the water from the garlic, leaving all of the garlic's therapeutic properties intact.

Pulped garlic was applied to pads of sphagnum moss and used to treat soldiers' wounds during World War I. You can try liquidising garlic with water and applying this to clean gauze as an antiseptic dressing, or combining it with vinegar for a cleansing — although stinging! — wash. It may also be used externally as a dressing for earache and toothache. Calluses, corns and bunions are common foot problems which are worsened by activity. Try rubbing the horny dead tissue with a crushed clove of garlic and slice of lemon; alternatively, bind them on with a bandage to soften and heal.

A douche made by combining 1 crushed garlic clove with 100 g of natural acidophilus yoghurt will effectively clear cystitis, often the result of the increased vaginal secretions experienced during pregnancy or unusual exertion, especially during unseasonably hot or humid weather. Garlic is a tried and true remedy for almost all internal infections. So if you are prone to recurrent gastrointestinal upsets or vaginal infections like candidiasis, try drinking garlic tea four times a day, using 2 or 3 mashed cloves to a mug of boiling water. If you find the strong aroma objectionable, look for odourless freeze-dried garlic. Another tip to remember is that the odour of garlic can be countered by chewing parsley or mint leaves.

Tip:

Include more garlic in your diet — it's a wonderful skin food because it's rich in sulphur compounds, which provide an instant skin boost and cleanse the system.

WINTER GARLIC SOUP

1 to 2 garlic bulbs, coarsely chopped

2 tsp olive oil

4 cups good quality chicken broth

2 to 4 egg yolks, beaten

½ cup dry red wine

Saute the chopped garlic in the olive oil until translucent and tender. It is not necessary to peel the individual cloves. Add the chicken broth. Bring to a slow boil, then reduce the heat and simmer gently until the garlic is mushy, about 30 minutes. Push through a strainer into a small pot. Add the beaten egg yolks slowly, stirring all the while. Return to the heat until thickened, add the wine slowly. Serves 4 to 6 people.

GERANIUM

An infusion of geranium (Pelargonium spp.) leaves and flowers has stimulating, soothing and healing properties. Used in the bath, it will help to heal minor irritations of the skin and reduce swellings. When added to bathwater in winter, it has the added bonus of promoting circulation and being warming to the skin. Use it as a base for preparing homemade beauty aids and skin fresheners. It is particularly indicated for dry or dehydrated skin, for poor circulation and as a general 'soother'.

Geranium is also wonderfully fragrant and essential oil of geranium is often included in commercial health and beauty preparations as a good blending aromatic. Folklore has it that this herb was an aphrodisiac, its warming and pleasant scent supposedly overcoming problems of frigidity.

Tip:

A ginger compress on the forehead (made by soaking a face cloth in the cooled tea) will help relieve a headache due to the nausea of pregnancy.

GINGER

Try adding ginger (Zingiber officinale) tea to hot water for soaking a sprained ankle, then bind with hot apple cider vinegar compresses. Topical application of both these natural remedies helps boost circulation of blood to the affected area, thus speeding the healing process. Grated ginger is also effective as an internal tonic in treating heartburn. Add sparingly to food or herbal teas to relieve flatulence and indigestion. Take hot ginger tea to treat symptoms of a cold or flu, and to cleanse the system of toxins by encouraging perspiration. Ginger tablets and capsules are a useful food supplement for those plagued with faulty digestion or colic. Ginger is an important drug in traditional Chinese medicine, being respected as a tonic and stimulant to ease flatulence and prevent nausea, as well as an antispasmodic to treat cramping, such as menstrual pain.

Tip:

Ginger also promotes circulation and is warming in winter time: try soaking feet for 15 minutes in a bowl of hot water to which 1 teaspoon of powdered ginger has been added.

GINSENG

Ginseng (Panax ginseng) powder will help regulate the body temperature as it is an 'alterative' or 'body restorer'. Use as the Chinese do — add it to chicken soup to help restore ill patients to health. Overcome fatigue with a cup of ginseng tea. This acts as a body and glandular balancer, and energises the whole body because it stimulates the adrenals and spleen. Chew the fresh or dried root, or add a pinch of the extract to food when cooking, to help regulate temperature imbalances and dizziness during hot weather. Ginseng is also available in tablet form or in capsules.

Recent research has shown that the active ingredients of ginseng produce an insulin-like effect against diabetes while the so-called phenolic compounds — salicylic acid, vanillic acid and syringic acid — have an apparent anti-ageing effect through the inhibition of lipid peroxide formation, thus slowing down tissue destruction and the degeneration of the cell membranes. Other intriguing scientific research points to ginseng as being of benefit in treating liver disorders, reducing blood cholesterol levels, bolstering the immune system, and even in suppressing the growth of cancerous tumours.

GLA (GAMMA LINOLEIC ACID)

See Evening Primrose Oil.

GLYCERINE

Glycerine is a thickened, sticky, sweetish-tasting clear liquid which is derived from vegetable oils. It is sometimes used as an ingredient in health preparations, notably tonics and demulcent syrups for the gastrointestinal tract, for its soothing properties. It is probably better known as an ingredient in natural beauty preparations, both as a moisturiser and a skin softener. Being plant derived, it is favoured by 'cruelty-free' cosmetic companies that neither test their products on animals nor use any ingredients, such as collagen and elastin, which are derived from by-products of animal slaughter.

GOLDENSEAL

After tooth extraction, put a few drops of boiling water on a goldenseal (*Hydrastis canadensis*) tea bag. Tap some extra goldenseal powder (to obtain, split open a capsule containing the powder) on this and place it over the wound to reduce swelling, pain and bleeding. This herb has a positive effect on skin tissue and on the mucous membranes and may be used for many skin disorders as well as for mouth ulcers, sore eyes and catarrh.

Tip:

Goldenseal is an excellent herb to use for undereye puffiness. Either place cooled wet tea bags on the eyes, or make an infusion from the powdered herb (½ teaspoon to 1 cup of hot water), strain and use to bathe the eyes.

Drink a mild tea of goldenseal and honey if beset by nausea, indigestion or frequent flatulence. Prepare the tea with a pinch of goldenseal powder in a cup of hot water; add honey to overcome the bitter taste. The goldenseal plant is native to North America, and years ago, the Native Americans used goldenseal tea as a tonic for gastric and liver disorders, as a laxative and to counter the nausea of morning sickness, then passing this knowledge on to the early settlers.

GOOSEBERRY

Gooseberries (*Ribes grossularia* and R. *divaricatum*) are a good source of vitamins A and C, as well as thiamine, potassium, phosphorus, iron, niacin and riboflavin. Vitamin C is now being explored in scientific research for its benefits in treating infections. Perhaps this use is not so new, though, when we see what herbalist John Gerard had to say in the 16th century about vitamin C-rich gooseberries: 'The juyce of the greene Gooseberries, cooleth all inflamations, Erysipelas and Saint Anthonie's fire'.

In Gerard's time, gooseberry leaves were also used in salads and as a natural remedy for expelling toxins and clearing sluggish blood in springtime, much as dandelion greens were and still are. A long-lived descendant of this practice is the Kentish children's traditional snack of young gooseberry leaves, which they call 'bread and cheese'.

GOOSEGRASS

You may see this listed as an ingredient in a natural deodorant or body spray. An infusion of the leaves is healing, gently astringent and has deodorant properties. It is particularly useful for oily skin, which needs regular cleansing to prevent blocked pores that develop into spots, blackheads or infected, reddened areas.

HAWTHORN

Anxiety associated with high blood pressure should be treated by a qualified herbalist and the condition supervised by a doctor. A herbalist will probably prescribe a combination of hawthorn (*Crataegus oxyacantha*) berries and lime flowers, with certain other herbs which you may need. Hawthorn berries are very effective in increasing the muscular action of the heart and are used to treat angina, palpitations, irregular pulse and other circulatory disorders. Hawthorn berries may also eliminate some types of heart-rhythm disturbances, or arrhythmias.

Hawthorn is widely used in German medicine, where herbs are more widely accepted as part of mainstream medicine. There, doctors readily prescribe 1 teaspoon of hawthorn tincture twice a day in the treatment of angina and congestive heart conditions. Lower potency versions, also based on hawthorn berries, are available in your health food store. Two cups of hawthorn tea, each made from 2 teaspoons of the dried crushed leaves and berries, may be drunk per day as part of a heart health program. Hawthorn tea is also a useful natural remedy for insomnia and, being a diuretic, may assist in maintaining kidney health.

HENNA

Probably the oldest known cosmetic colouring agent is henna (*Lawsonia inermis*). Mummified remains from Egyptian tombs show that a mixture of henna and indigo shoots, called *henna reng*, was used to colour hair and beards to a youthful blue-black. The leaves of henna are sold dried and ground to a dark brown powder and are used in Eastern countries to dye the hands and feet. Henna was also used by the prophet Mohammed to dye his beard.

Henna is very versatile. It can be mixed with other organic substances to modify the colour — coffee, wine, eggs, lemon juice and onion skins are modern variations. Henna essence and henna extract both appear often on all manner of natural hair preparations and colorants. It does not necessarily mean that the product will dye the hair — 'clear' henna is a marvellous hair conditioner and nourishing treatment, helping to smooth hair shafts roughened through commercial treatments such as perming, and to reduce split ends and fragile hair conditions.

Traditionalists might wish to experiment with the pure henna powder by adding dried indigo shoots, walnut husks and lucerne (darkening) or betel nuts (reddening). It is important to test the effect of both your own henna mixture or a purchased one on a small piece of hair before dyeing, as it can 'take' a lot more rapidly than pharmaceutical brands! The great advantage of henna is that the hair is thoroughly conditioned as it is being dyed, the henna giving each hair strength, body and lustre.

Tip:

Try henna as an alternative to nail varnish, which can cause yellowing of the nails. Mix up the paste according to the manufacturer's directions and apply it to clean, dry nails, and leave to dry in the sun or by the fire, for any warmth will intensify the colour. When dry, buff the nails to a high polish and they will have a soft apricot tint.

HONEY

The ancient Egyptians looked upon bees and their honey as the source of eternal life and health. Honey was used by the priests who were charged with the sacred tasks of embalming and mummification and it was also widely employed as a food preservative. Legend has it that Jupiter, the chief god in Roman

Tip:

For a refreshing facial, try honey with your favourite fruit. Mix 1 tablespoon of raw honey with 1 teaspoon of olive oil, 1 egg yolk and 1 tablespoon fresh fruit pulp. Try apple (softens skin and acts as an astringent), pear (a super moisturiser), orange (has great softening powers), rockmelon (rehydrates dry skin), strawberry (tones, softens and moisturises) or banana (soothes, softens and smooths).

mythology, transformed the beautiful nymph Melissa into a bee so that she could prepare the miracle substance for healing. And, in recent times, honey has been successfully tested as a healing agent in scientific laboratories as well as hospitals.

Honey is a natural healer. It has high prophylactic properties that help to halt or control the ageing process, and because of its high vitamin and potassium content, it nourishes the skin, promotes moisture retention, prevents and erases wrinkles and helps to treat skin eruptions. To test this, soak small pads of cotton wool in raw honey and place them over skin eruptions such as acne. Repeat often, especially after washing. Leave on overnight if possible. Or apply honey to gauze and wrap this dressing over blemishes. Renew daily until eruptions disappear.

Here's a hand cream formula that is adapted from a very old Hebrew recipe. It also works wonders on sunburned skin.

Tip:

Dry flaky skin on the feet is a common complaint. In addition to keeping feet well moisturised, try the following honey-based treatment. Splash warm water on feet, rub in a good layer of honey and leave for half an hour to be well absorbed by the skin. Rinse off the honey with warm water and pat dry. Use the remedy daily until the condition improves.

HONEY HAND CREAM

2 tablespoons raw honey
1 cup thick yoghurt
contents of 1 vitamin A capsule

Combine all ingredients thoroughly, whizzing together in a blender till smooth; refrigerate before and after use.

HOPS

Hops are the cone-like flowers borne by the climbing hop vine (*Humulus lupulus*) and are probably most famous for the part they play in beer making. However, they also have applications in the world of natural health and beauty. An oil from the plant is used in colognes and perfumes and dried hops have been much used through the ages to soothe the nerves and induce sleep. Dried hops are also much used in herbal bath preparations and facial masks. Hops or hop oil is used by herbalists as a sedative and as an antispasmodic digestive aid. The plant's sedative prowess is due to the presence of a potent chemical, 2-methyl–3-butene–2-ol, which actually becomes stronger as it is dried, so use aged dried hops for best effect. In fact, they are an age-old remedy for sleeplessness. A charming recipe from Ram's *Little Dodoen*, a 17th century manuscript for ladies, instructs the insomniac to 'Take dried Rose leaves, hops, powder of mints, powder of cloves . . . then put all these together in a bag and take that to bed with you and it will cause you to sleep, and it is good to smell unto at other times'.

Tip:

Insomnia can be helped by using equal quantities of lime flowers, hops and lemon balm in a warm decoction to take before going to bed. Some people find a small sleep-pillow stuffed with hops very effective too.

HORSE CHESTNUT

Occasionally, you will see essence of horse chestnut (*Aesculus hippocastanum*) listed as an ingredient in bath or natural beauty care products. The seeds of this tree contain tannin, and when infused, they make an astringent, health-promoting liquid which is wonderfully stimulating. It is popular for use in after-bath gels, body lotions and cooling creams for acne. Being an astringent and tonic herb, it may also be used to treat inflammatory skin conditions or problems such as varicose veins, haemorrhoids, diarrhoea and fevers.

HORSERADISH

Armoracia rusticana, as it is officially known, was originally a native of eastern Europe. It is one of the 'five bitter herbs' said to have been eaten by the ancient Hebrews during their eight days of Passover. (The others were coriander, horehound, lettuce and nettle.) Prescribed since mediaeval days as a medicinal herb, horseradish's use as an antiscorbutic (vitamin C supplement) is ancient and remains valid. Better yet, horseradish is a member of the *Cruciferae* family, which cancer societies worldwide have cited for its anticarcinogenic properties. Grating horseradish releases a volatile oil rich in blood-stabilising sulphur. The pungent aroma means that, unsurprisingly, this herb is a marvellous natural remedy for all sinus-related complaints, notably congestion and infection.

Tip:

To make a power-packed tonic to clear a congested head, juice enough fresh, peeled and cubed horseradish root to produce about ¼ cup liquid. Combine this with approximately 4 cups of a vegetable juice of your preference, say, tomato. Serve warm or over ice.

HORSETAIL

To make a valuable tonic rinse for the hair, prepare an infusion of horsetail (*Equisetum arvense*) and sage. This will add lustre to the hair and enhance its natural colour. Horsetail is also considered a baldness cure. While I cannot guarantee that this herb will actually persuade a bald pate to sprout luscious new hair, tradition insists it does. Since hair and nails are formed from the same substance — keratin — horsetail is also thought to be of great benefit to nails. Soak fragile or easily split nails and cuticles in a strong tea made from horsetail (25 g to 500 ml water) every night for a fortnight and you will see definite

Tip:

HORSETAIL SKIN CLEANSER
This is especially suitable for teenagers with excessively oily skin. Combine 2 tablespoons of strong horsetail tea with enough oatmeal to form a pasty consistency, and smooth onto clean, damp skin. Allow to remain for up to 5 minutes, then rinse off with tepid water and pat dry with a soft towel. Similarly, horsetail tea may be diluted with distilled water and used as a skin tonic for normal to oily skin.

improvements. This tea would make a good astringent wash for inflamed skin, or a mouthwash for gum inflammations or ulcers, too. Horsetail tea is a powerful diuretic and may be prescribed for kidney or bladder problems. It also has tonic and stimulant properties for the blood, and is helpful for anaemia. Horsetail tablets and capsules are also available.

HOUSELEEK

A decoction or tincture made from the leaves of the tiny houseleek (*Sempervivum tectorum*) is healing and nourishing; it is a useful addition to moisturising creams and lotions if your skin needs constant care to replace missing natural oils. It is an emollient and astringent herb and so may also be used in gentle cleansers. Old-style gardeners may refer to it as 'hen-and-chickens'. Pick the fresh leaves, crush lightly and use to ease the pain of insect bites or stings. The juice from the snapped-open leaves is thought to have healing properties for haemorrhoids, corns and warts, too.

HYSSOP

Hyssop (*Hyssopus officinalis*) is a useful household plant and may be used to scent rooms and notepaper and to add colour and fragrance to potpourri. The flowers can be ground and used as an effective strong-tasting tooth powder or for refreshing aromatic baths, which also have a positive effect on muscular stiffness or aches. Centuries ago, herbalist Nicolas Culpeper wrote that hyssop 'boiled with wine, [is] good to take away inflammations [and] the blue and black marks that come by strokes, bruises and falls'. Alternatively, look for the essential oil and experiment with it as a beauty steam or an inhalation. Hyssop oil is astringent and tonic, having a stimulating effect on the skin and body when added to bath preparations.

The following recipe, 'To Make a Bath for Melancholy', appeared in the 17th century manuscript, 'Arcana Fairfaxiana'. 'Take Mallowes, pellitory of the Wall, of each three handfuls, Camomell flowers, Melilot flowers, of each one handful; hollyhocks, two handfuls, Isop [Hyssop] one great handful, Senerick seed one ounce, and boil them in nine gallons of Water until they come to three, then put in a quart of new milke and go into it bloud warm or something warmer.'

Hyssop tea or syrup can be used for sore throats and catarrh, a cooled diluted tea is a cooling and refreshing eyebath, while the crushed leaves may be placed directly onto wounds to promote healing.

IRISH MOSS

You may see this listed as an ingredient in many differ-ent brands of cosmetics, skin tonics and emollient creams now that 'full ingredients disclosure' is the norm amongst manufacturing companies, and you may won-der what a seaweed (which is what it is) is doing there! Irish moss (*Chondrus crispus*) is a highly nutritive seaweed from the British Isles which looks like a moss, hence the name. It is also called carrageen. Irish moss is an effec-tive and inexpensive stabiliser and emollient in creams and lotions, as well as being a useful emollient in its own right. It can be made into a nourishing jelly high in minerals and sulphur compounds, with demulcent, moisturising and emollient effects on the skin.

IRON

It has been shown that people whose diets are low in iron or who have absorption problems may lose their hair. They may also experience mood swings, lethargy, dizziness and a feeling of perpetual exhaustion. Sixty-five per cent of the functioning iron in the body is found in haemoglobin, the principal component of red blood cells. Haemoglobin acts as a carrier of oxygen from the lungs to the tissues, which die if deprived of oxygen.

Iron positively affects the production of T-cells, the key participants in our immune systems. Candida and herpes simplex infections are both more common in individuals who are iron-deficient. Iron is especially important for a new mother, both to have sufficient levels herself and to consider breastfeeding, because iron-related immunity is conferred through human breast milk.

Although some of the processed foods we eat today

are 'fortified' with iron, it is not in the form most easily absorbed. It is best to eat a nutritious diet of lean meat, fish, legumes, dried fruit, whole grains and dark green, leafy vegetables.

If intestinal absorption is impaired, taking digestive enzymes is indicated (ask your health food store or pharmacist). Take iron supplements only under the supervision of a nutritionist or doctor. Taking vitamin C along with the iron enhances its absorption.

IVY

Ivy (Hedera spp.) extract or ivy essence is listed as an ingredient in many beauty preparations, skin creams and tonics, especially exfoliating pastes for the face and body. It does have a noticeable effect on cellulite, helping to break down fatty deposits and improve the circulation of the blood to the skin's surface, thus helping to rid the circulatory system of the toxins which build up and cause cellulite in the first place. The plant itself may be employed as a natural remedy — take 1 cupful of ivy (leaves and stalks only, the berries are poisonous) and boil in enough water to cover for 15 minutes. Remove from heat and allow to cool slightly, then strain through a nonmetallic strainer, pressing down well on the plant material to extract the essence. Soak cotton pads in the lukewarm liquid and use on body areas affected by cellulite. To use, either massage liquid directly into skin or, if time allows, loosely bind pads soaked in the liquid to the areas and leave for 20 minutes whilst lying down. An ivy-based poultice is a useful natural remedy for boils, ulcers, sores and all manner of other skin problems. A tincture of ivy leaves was once a respected treatment for whooping cough.

Tip:

Try ivy compresses for swollen ankles during pregnancy, or bathe feet and ankles in warm ivy 'tea', as made above.

JASMINE

Jasmine (*Jasminum officinalis*) has one of the most aromatic and sensual of fragrances, and an infusion made from jasmine or jessamine tea or from the essential oil is wonderfully fragrant and uplifting. Jasmine is much used in perfumery production as a blending scent and in many natural beauty preparations based on the principles of aromatherapy. As well as offering its superb fragrance, jasmine oil has a noted smoothing and moisturising effect on the skin and hair, helping to soften and heal in much the same way as rose oil. Essential oil of jasmine is used by professional aromatherapists as an aphrodisiac, as an antidepressant, to speed up labour, for postnatal depression, to treat respiratory problems and menstrual pain, and as a general 'pep up'. The berries are poisonous, but it is interesting to note that a homoeopathic tincture made from them is prescribed for convulsions and blood poisoning.

JOJOBA

Jojoba (*Simmondsia californica*) is pronounced 'ho-ho-ba' and is a desert shrub. The fruit of the female plant produces seed kernels about the size of a peanut, which, when pressed, impart an extremely pure oil. The oil is similar in characteristics to the oil of the now protected sperm whale. It has become one of the single most sought-after natural remedies today, being used increasingly in many skin and hair preparations. The quality that has made it most desirable is its ability to be absorbed readily through several layers of skin, providing softness without greasiness.

Jojoba oil has been touted as the miracle cure for most hair problems ranging from baldness to dandruff. Because of its similarity to sebum, the protective oil produced by your skin and scalp, it does have a positive effect on many hair-related problems. Jojoba oil has been found to help remove sebum which has become embedded at the base of the hair. This oil plug 'chokes' the hair strand, interfering with its health or even preventing it from growing at all. When the embedded sebum is freed, hair can grow normally again, and with a renewed layer of oil flowing over the scalp, certain types of dandruff or scaling are stopped altogether while hair takes on a healthy rejuvenated shine. Another interesting effect of jojoba is that it appears to soothe an 'angry' scalp, progressively diminishing excess sebaceous secretions, redness and flaking of the scalp. Jojoba meal, made from the flesh of the bean after it has been pressed to create jojoba oil, has very gentle exfoliant properties and is highly absorbent; it is a common base ingredient in body scrubs and cleansing masks.

JUNIPER

Juniper (*Juniperus communis*) berries are used to produce an essence which is a traditional natural remedy for kidney infections, having a pronounced diuretic and antiseptic effect. Due to this water-emitting action, juniper is also indicated for gout and rheumatism and for stomach problems that are caused by internal congestions, such as colic and flatulence. It has an antiseptic effect and stimulates the circulation, thereby assisting to clear skin problems. Use externally by adding a few drops of essential oil of juniper to a bath before going to bed for its calming and relaxing properties and to help heal any skin irritations. Use internally by adding 2 to 3 drops to a glass of water and taking this for indigestion. Two to three drops of juniper oil in a steam inhalation are a useful natural remedy for bronchitis and other lung disorders.

Tip:

Juniper berries and shoots, when infused in bathwater, can help to relieve aching joints. Alternatively, add 5 to 6 drops of juniper essential oil to warm bathwater.

KAOLIN

Kaolin comes from the Chinese words for high hill. It is a powdered natural hydrated aluminium silicate — put simply, this means it is a fine white clay. Though insoluble, it is often listed as an ingredient in natural face masks and exfoliating products because of its power to absorb moisture; it is also used to bind cosmetic preparations. When mixed with water it makes a soft smooth paste with exfoliant effects.

KELP

Venus came from the sea, and perhaps the old Romans knew a thing or two, since 'beauty from the sea' comes in the form of the high-mineral contents of fish and — seaweed! The long ribbons of the kelp or bladderwrack plant (*Fucus vesiculosus*) grow in huge oceanic forests off the coast of the Atlantic ocean and the Baltic, Irish and North seas, and have many potent restorative properties. Both are beneficial to your diet and health and therefore to your skin and hair quality and overall sense of wellbeing. Kelp is a mineral-rich health supplement and acts as a gentle tonic for the metabolism and as a thyroid restorative. Herbalists may prescribe kelp for low thyroid activity and other symptoms of a sluggish constitution. (Sea water, interestingly, has a similar composition to human blood, and swimming regularly in unpolluted sea water will almost certainly improve your complexion, as well as your muscle tone.)

Tip:

Mix kelp powder with fruit juice. This will provide a potent skin-saving drink, rich in the iron, iodine, trace minerals and nutrients your skin needs.

For those who want an 'easier way', kelp tablets and powder offer these naturally occurring minerals in a highly concentrated form. Kelp powder and granules are also sometimes listed as ingredients in 'savoury salts' or salt substitutes and, of course, kelp is an ingredient of

Japanese cuisine. Remember, whilst salty sea water is good for you externally, refined common salt is toxic in excess quantities and is a contributing factor in hypertension and fluid retention. Be in the swim with a low salt diet and avoid periodic puffiness.

Tip:

Add kelp powder to your bathwater; it can be marvellously restorative to the skin.

KIWI FRUIT

The Chinese gooseberry (*Actinidia chinensis*), commonly known as kiwi fruit, has never really enjoyed popularity in its homeland and it was not used in cookery there at all, let alone for any medicinal purposes. About the only compliment the Chinese paid this fruit was that it was particularly thirst-quenching.

In fact, kiwi fruit are useful as a natural remedy, as well as being favourite decorative fruit and a taste treat in their own right. Kiwi fruit are a good source of vitamin A, iron, some potassium and phosphorus, and have a higher vitamin C content than most citrus fruits. This makes them excellent first foods for recuperating patients, babies or sick children. Interestingly, kiwi fruit are an excellent tenderiser for meats and may be eaten with a tough cut of steak or pork to make it more palatable and digestible.

LADY'S MANTLE

The leaves of lady's mantle or lion's foot (*Alchemilla vulgaris*) are healing, astringent and reduce inflammation. The leaves and stems are rich in naturally occurring tannins, meaning this herb has a potent astringent and styptic action. It may be used externally as a skin tonic or for wounds or discharging wounds; internally, it may be useful as a natural remedy for excessive menstrual bleeding and as a digestive tonic to improve the appetite, to stop diarrhoea and to strengthen the heart and blood vessels. An infusion or tincture made from this herb will have tonic and cleansing properties and will be best suited to recipes or products which cater for oily skin which needs regular cleansing. A tea made from 1 to 4 g of the dried herb, taken up to three times a day, is useful as a douche for vaginal discharges, sores or infections. For centuries, it has been used for this purpose, earning the nickname 'lady's best friend'. It was also traditionally used as a drink after childbirth, to help stem any internal bleeding.

Tip:

Most people have some oily areas of skin on their face, and blackheads and whiteheads tend to congregate where there is an excess of grease. Beaten egg white combined with an infusion of lady's mantle — made by infusing 2 tablespoons of the dried herb in a glass and a half of boiling water — is recommended for clearing excessively oily skin.

LANOLIN

Lanolin is a rich, sticky, fatty paste extracted from sheep's wool. It is a very old-fashioned — but nonetheless extremely effective — moisturiser and healing agent for cuts, chapped skin, nicks and nappy rash. It is an invaluable ingredient in all manner of creams and lotions as it is so easily absorbed by the skin. If you are preparing your own homemade recipes, look for anhydrous lanolin as this is prepared without water and you will be able to enjoy the maximum beneficial effect of the lanolin.

LAVENDER

Lavender (*Lavandula vera*) has long been cultivated for its scent. In his *Livre des Parfums* of 1864, Eugene Rimmel described it as 'a nice clean scent and an old and deserving favourite'. Commercial perfume houses still use it as the basic ingredient of many fragrances and as an additive to cologne, *chypre* and leather varieties. In addition, its very soothing, anti-septic and anti-inflammatory properties mean this well-loved flower — specifical-ly the pure essence or oil — may be used to make a variety of natural beauty aids and remedies.

Tip:

Lavender water is very useful for reducing scalp oiliness. Soak a piece of cloth in a basin of strong lavender tea and rub through the hair to trap dirt and grime.

Lavender oil may be used to make an effective mouthwash, skin tonic and eye lotion, and helps to treat mild infections or irritations, such as cuts, insect bites and fun-gal infections. Try a few drops in the bath to heal skin troubled by a rash. To scent the skin and stimulate the circulation, combine lavender oil with other scented oils from its own plant family, such as marjoram and rosemary, and an unscented carrier oil such as apricot kernel oil. The essence will also blend well with gerani-um and rose.

Lavender oil helps to regenerate skin cells and so is excellent for burns — especially sunburn — and for chapping. Also, by balancing the activity of the seba-ceous glands, products containing lavender oil or essence will tone oily skin and help to treat acne. If you are plagued by a nasty pimple, take a cotton bud and dab it firstly in camphor, then in lavender oil, before applying directly to the blemish. This will often, miraculously, clear up the culprit overnight.

Lavender is also well known as a headache herb: made into a weak tea (1 teaspoon of dried herb to 600 ml of boiling water), it may be dabbed on the temples and forehead or used as a refreshing facial rinse.

AROMATIC LAVENDER BATH OIL

15 ml oil of lavender
2 ml oil of thyme
500 ml 80 proof vodka
50 ml glycerine
200 ml distilled water

Combine all ingredients in a clear glass jar or bottle, cap securely and shake thoroughly before adding 1 to 2 table-spoons to a bath filled with warm water.

LECITHIN

Lecithin is available in either granule or powder form, or packaged in capsules or tablets. Lecithin is a phosphatide, containing choline and inositol, and acts as an emulsifying agent. Its presence in the blood tends to dissolve cholesterol and actually reduce the size of lipid or fat particles in the bloodstream. Some lecithin is manufactured by the body itself and a lot can be found in very ordinary foods such as nuts, vegetable oils and egg yolks. Other good food sources are seeds, whole-wheat cereal, wheat germ, soya bean oil and unrefined foods containing vegetable oils. In addition to its use as a food supplement, lecithin granules and powder are excellent bases for preparing natural cosmetics, being a natural emulsifier.

HONEY AND LECITHIN BRACER (FOR THE FEET)

1 *tablespoon each of avocado, olive and sesame oil*

1 *teaspoon liquid lecithin*

2 *tablespoons raw honey*

4 *teaspoons dried mint leaves*

Puree all ingredients in a blender until the mixture is quite smooth. Add 1 capful to a warm footbath and soak feet for 15 minutes or more. Rinse off with tepid water and pat dry with a soft towel.

Tip:

Don't throw away any squeezed-out lemon halves. Turned inside-out and dipped in sugar, you can use them, mitt-style, on roughened ankles or elbows, before rinsing and applying cold cream.

LEMON

The lemon (*Citrus limon*) has a long traditional use as a medicine. The Romans dosed pregnant women with lemon cordials, according to Pliny the Elder, 'to stay flux and vomit'. The lemon's antiseptic properties are well respected. The pulp is effective as a poultice to staunch bleeding and, blended with other female tonic herbs, may be prescribed during menstruation to reduce an excessive flow of bleeding. The juice makes an excellent gargle for a sore throat. It also has a mild sedative action and will thus reduce fever, as well as promoting bile activity and therefore easing any indigestion.

The lemon's medicinal claim to fame is, however, its use in treating scurvy, which caused the tragic deaths of early sea-voyagers. Even today, English sailors are required by law to drink a glass of lemon juice daily when at sea. Lemons are most important as a rich source of vitamin C and the bioflavonoids, which maintain the health of the skin's collagen content and strengthen the tiny capillaries seen near the surface of the

Tip:

If you find your face becomes oilier as the thermometer goes higher, squeeze the juice of half a lemon into a cup of water. Saturate cotton balls with this solution, chill and apply to nose and forehead for instant shine control.

skin. So they should be eaten for maximum natural health and beauty benefit, as well as applied to the skin or hair as a natural cosmetic.

Tip:
To refine and even out a splotchy tan, blend the juice of 1 lemon with ¼ cup of whole milk. Spread liberally over tanned areas, leave for 20 minutes, then rinse well with cool water.

Lemon juice has wonderful toning effects, mild deodorant properties and will provide a gentle exfoliant action. Use it in many ways — as a hair rinse, in baths to whiten the skin or bleach freckles, as an antibacterial dandruff treatment and a refreshing tooth cleanser. It is also excellent as a lotion to soothe a sunburned nose or shoulders.

Tip:
Mix lemon juice with cider vinegar, then stir through warm bathwater. Or hang a bath bag containing a tablespoon each of crushed dried lemon peel and fresh or dried rosemary leaves under the tap. As the water sluices through, enjoy the refreshing fragrance.

LEMON BALM

Lemon balm (*Melissa officinalis*) is native to the mountains of southern Europe, although for centuries now it has naturalised over much of the northern hemisphere. It has long been a favourite cottage garden plant and remains as popular among herbalists and natural therapists as a remedy as it was when the ancient Greek physician Dioscorides used lemon balm in wine to treat nervous disorders. A very old belief is that lemon balm causes merriment and relaxation. The 11th century Arab physician Avicenna wrote that 'Balm causeth the mind and the heart to become merry'. In the 17th century, Nicolas Culpeper was to agree, writing 'It [balm] causeth the mind and heart to become merry, and driveth away the troublesome care and thoughts arising from melancholy'.

John Gerard waxed very enthusiastic about lemon balm in his influential 16th century herbal, saying 'Bawme drunk in wine is good against the bitings of venomous beasts, comforts the heart and driveth away all melancholy and sadness'. In addition to its time-honoured use as a relaxing tea, he recommended it as a natural remedy for just about every ailment imaginable, from insomnia to arthritis. More recently, folk medicine tells us that lemon balm is thought to confer longevity on those who use it. A certain John Hussey, of Sydenham, England, attributed achieving his grand old age of 116 to having taken lemon balm tea, sweetened with honey, every day for 50 years.

Tip:

Crushed fresh lemon balm may be applied to a wound or graze as an emergency first aid measure, having a very mild antiseptic action.

Lemon balm contains volatile citrus oils which do have a powerful calming effect on the central nervous system. A tea is particularly good for smoothing out digestive disorders and tension and is very good for children's troubles, such as nausea or toothache. Recent research in Germany has confirmed lemon balm's traditional use as a digestive herb, proving that it does actually serve to relax the smooth muscle tissue of the digestive tract. A cup of lemon balm tea taken last thing at night will help a patient with a cold or the flu to get a good night's sleep. It will also help allay menstrual pains.

Tip:

Use lemon balm and marigold flowers and leaves as bath bag additives to relax tense, overworked muscles.

For a relaxing bath, tie a handful of fresh or dried lemon balm in a handkerchief and tie it to the hot water tap. As the hot bathwater sluices through the bag the refreshing aroma will be released.

LEMON GRASS

A useful and fragrant essential oil, lemon grass (*Cymbopogon citratus*) may be used to heal blemished skin, oily skin and sensitive skin; it is also indicated for easing aches and pains, healing burns and wounds, and for headaches, insomnia and depression. It has astringent and antiseptic properties and is a mild diuretic; some aromatherapists claim that, used in facial steams and all-over body saunas, lemon grass has age-retardant properties. Perhaps this is because lemon grass is rich in vitamin A, the 'skin vitamin'.

LETTUCE

Lactuca sativa refers to the most usual variety of garden lettuce; a great many new and fashionable varieties exist as well, such as the varicoloured mignonettes and the upright 'heart-less' cos. The juice of lettuce has long been employed as an astringent and cosmetic; pulped lettuce leaves are very soothing and cooling to the skin when used on the face as a mask, or sieved and added to the bath. Centuries ago, herbalist Nicolas Culpeper wrote of lettuce that 'The juyce . . . boyled with oyle of roses, applied to the Forehead and temples, procures sleep'. Indeed, lettuce tea is a surprisingly tasty and very effective natural sleep remedy.

LILY OF THE VALLEY

In his *New Herbal* of 1578, Henry Lyte called the lily of the valley 'the Lily Convall with flowers as white as snow and of pleasant strong savour. The water of the flowers comforteth the hearte . . . and doth strengthen the memorie.' Other herbalists over time have claimed a tincture of the flowers of lily of the valley (*Convallaria majalis*) would regulate a disturbed heartbeat and, quite recently, this remedy was used for treating British soldiers who had been subjected to nerve gas in World War I.

Tincture and essence of lily of the valley may be prescribed by a qualified herbalist in certain instances to a patient. It contains cardioactive glycosides, which means it can have a digitalis-like stimulating action on the contraction of the heart, increasing myocardial efficiency. However, instructions should *always* be followed strictly and self-medication of this herb is not recommended. More commonly, its perfumed essence is included in soaps, cosmetics and toiletries.

LIME FLOWERS (LINDEN)

It is reassuring to know time-honoured remedies may be used with confidence to deal with irritating aches and pains.

Tip:
An infusion of lime blossoms may be added to bathwater; it is marvellous for soothing frayed nerves.

Lime flower (Tilia europaea) tea quiets the nerves and promotes sleep, while a pillow stuffed with the dried flowers is an old-fashioned way of ensuring an undisturbed night. These methods are also recommended for soothing irritable or colicky babies. A tea made from lime flowers is a gentle but effective relaxant for anxious or irritable children, perhaps around exam time. A herbalist may prescribe a higher dosage — up to 4 g of the dried flowers three or more times a day — as a peripheral vasodilator in the treatment of a patient with hypertension or atherosclerosis problems. It is also an important remedy in treating a fever.

LIME FLOWER MASSAGE OIL
2 handfuls dried lime flowers
200 ml avocado oil
100 ml apple cider vinegar

Pack flowers into a clean glass jar, cover with oil and cap securely. Leave in a cool, dark place for 3 weeks, shaking occasionally to ensure flowers are covered. Pour off the mixture into a non-aluminium saucepan, heat until medium-warm, then remove from heat, strain off the flowers and add the cider vinegar to the oil. Pour into a sterilised jar, cool and cap. Shake thoroughly before use and store in refrigerator between uses.

LINSEED

See Flax.

LIQUORICE

Liquorice (*Glycyrrhiza glabra*) is a perennial shrub which grows up to 1.25 metres high. The root is cultivated and harvested for use as a natural remedy: the powdered root is used in cough syrups and linctuses, tonics for the digestion, and syrups or tablets for treating constipation. The sweet, spicy oil is used in aromatherapy for soothing the skin and to refresh and soothe the nerves. The powdered root is also a common ingredient in natural cosmetics, especially toothpastes or powders and gargles, being included to reduce inflammation and for its astringent effect on gums as well as for its flavour. Herbalists may prescribe a stronger dosage — up to 4 g of the dried root or its equivalent in capsules, tablets or a decoction three times a day — for gastric ulcers or other internal inflammatory conditions. (Caution: it should not be used therapeutically by patients with hypertension problems as it can tend to increase fluid retention and blood pressure.)

LOOFAH

Along with sponges, loofahs must be one of the most ancient beauty bath aids you could use. A sponge is the skeleton of a sea creature and tends to be softer and to hold a great deal more water. Loofahs are the fibrous matrix of tropical gourds, and being less soft than sponges, they make an excellent skin brush for elbows, knees, feet and any other rough surfaces of the skin. As loofahs hold less water than sponges, they dry more quickly and so can be used regularly as a gentle exfoliant, toning the skin and ridding it of the dead skin cell layer. Use your loofah with caution, however, particularly if your skin is very soft and sensitive. Soak it well before using it for the first time and be very gentle if you apply it to the face.

LOVAGE

Lovage (*Levisticum officinale*) was very popular in Britain and was grown in early monastic herb gardens, more for medicinal use than as a potherb. Ninth century Swiss Benedictine monks — they of the liqueur fame! — prescribed an infusion of lovage for various disorders. It is a digestive herb and has a warming and soothing effect on gastrointestinal upsets as well as helping to remove flatulence. Lovage was also, and still is, a popular bath herb, being added to the bath for its fresh scent and notable cleansing and deodorising effect on the skin. Perhaps this also explains why it was once considered an aphrodisiac and love charm. Czechoslovakian girls would tuck small bags of lovage in their clothes when they were seeking a lover.

Tip:

Add 4 to 5 drops of essential oil of lovage to warm bathwater. Or make your own scented decoction to use in the bath by steeping 30 g of chopped, peeled lovage root in 300 ml of boiling water for 10 minutes, then allowing to cool and straining before use.

Lovage leaves or a decoction of lovage may both be used in the bath. Lovage is mildly antiseptic and antibacterial, so it makes a good gargle for a sore throat, too. Seventeenth century herbalist Nicolas Culpeper wrote that 'The distilled water helps the quinsy of the throat if the throat and the mouth be gargled with it, and it helps the pleurisy if drunk three or four times'.

With its digestive and antispasmodic properties, a cup of lovage tea makes a comforting and warming drink for infants with colicky digestive disturbances. A strong decoction of the roots may be used as a cleansing and mildly antiseptic dressing for wounds and grazes. A decoction made from the leaves is also a traditional beauty aid, being thought to bleach the skin and help remove pimples. And Culpeper also wrote that 'the distilled water of lovage takes away the redness and dimness of the eyes if dropped into them'.

MAGNESIUM

If, as a woman, you have monthly bouts of bad temper, you might suffer from periodic fluid retention, which literally creates pressure on your nerves and helps cause that notorious female crabbiness. A diet high in magnesium-containing foods is recommended — figs and dates score well here. Several tonics which contain magnesium along with vitamin B$_6$ are also helpful to the nervous system.

Magnesium may be taken to help poor circulation and complexion problems. Menstrual cramping may be relieved by a higher intake of magnesium along with additional calcium found in dairy foods and sesame seeds. Other good food sources include bran, honey, green vegetables, nuts, seafood, spinach, bonemeal and kelp. Some deficiency symptoms include nervousness, insomnia, twitchy eyelids and nervous squinting.

Current nutritional studies are focusing on magnesium as a major antidote to stress. Magnesium controls the level of other electrolytes, such as potassium, calcium and sodium, all of which are present in the fluid in which the muscles are bathed. Magnesium tends to relax and smooth muscles and dilate the arteries, while calcium and sodium tend to constrict arteries. Under stress, magnesium levels decline rapidly, leaving calcium and sodium more dominant. The smooth muscles may begin to tremble or go into spasm. Indications are that a magnesium deficiency focuses on vasoconstriction of arteries in the heart area, rather than throughout the body. Samples of heart muscle from heart attack victims reveal magnesium levels 10 to 35 per cent below normal.

Another role of magnesium is to stabilise platelet clumping in the blood. Any magnesium deficiency increases the ability of the platelet to clump and thus blocks a coronary artery, precipitating a heart attack. A magnesium deficiency also contributes to arterial fibrillation (irregular heartbeat) and to migraine headaches.

MARJORAM

The ancient Greeks and Romans used marjoram (*Origanum hortensis*) enthusiastically and gave it the nickname of 'joy of the mountains', as it was often found growing in wild, inhospitable or craggy areas. As well as being a popular culinary herb, used to flavour meat and cheese dishes, marjoram was also a common ingredient in 'sweete powderes, sweete bagges and sweete washyng waters', according to 16th century herbalist John Gerard.

Marjoram has been widely used for medicinal purposes. Early physicians used it as an antidote to poisoning, snake venom and hemlock. The Romans used marjoram tea widely for settling the stomach and for dizziness. Seventeenth century herbalist Nicolas Culpeper recommended marjoram as 'an excellent remedy for the braine and other parts of the body', adding that a dressing of powdered marjoram and honey would help reduce 'the marks of blows and bruises'.

Tip:

New information suggests that essential oil of marjoram may be used to reduce the spread of fungal and viral disorders, such as herpes, in much the same way as tea tree oil.

Marjoram tea has a soothing and calming effect on the nerves while the essential oil has mild antiseptic and tonic properties. Contemporary herbalists often recommend the tea as a digestive aid, or prescribe a strong infusion for a sore throat. The strongly aromatic oil may be added to a massage oil and used as a warming rub for muscular aches. Interesting new research shows that marjoram tea will also help to alleviate menstrual cramps and often bring on delayed menstruation in women: for this reason, pregnant women should obviously not use more than the culinary amount.

MARSH MALLOW

The marsh mallow plant (Althaea officinalis) has been renowned through the ages as a herb to soothe inflamed or sensitive skin. The root and leaves are emollient and healing. It may be used internally as a tea or in a syrup to soothe an upset stomach or any irritation of the gastrointestinal tract; it is also valuable as an ingredient in cough syrups to loosen a tight, dry cough or bronchial tension. Herbalists may prescribe a tincture of marsh mallow to soothe inflammations of the stomach or small intestine, such as gastritis or a peptic ulcer, or as a gentle curative for inflamed urinary passages, such as occur with cystitis or with urinary stones, as it is a mild diuretic. For external use, marsh mallow powder or tincture may be listed as an ingredient in fine light lotions, soap or cleanser. It is particularly appropriate for very fine skin types with insufficient surface oils.

MASKS

Masks have been a natural health and beauty aid since before Cleopatra applied Nile River clay to her face for a wrinkle-free, glowing skin. Tradition has it that the first such mask was invented by slave girls washing clothes at the river's edge. They found their feet, immersed in the mud, became soft and white, and so decided to use the same mud on their hands and faces.

As part of your natural health and beauty program, replace laboratory-designed 21st century masks with masks using natural ingredients. Here are two tried-and-true recipes.

For a tropical fruit mask with vitamin A, take crushed pineapple and crushed pawpaw (50:50) to make ½ cup of pulp and mix to a paste with wheat germ. Apply to clean dry skin and leave for 15 minutes before rinsing off.

These lush fruits are rich sources of the skin vitamins A and C, plus the skin-softening enzymes, bromelain and papain.

For a zingy whipped fruit mask, take 1 cup pulped fresh apricots (or soaked dried apricots, pureed), ½ cup mineral water and 1 tablespoon of raw honey. Mix in a blender, then apply over throat, face and shoulders. Apricots are full of essential oils, emollients and vitamin A. Honey is Mother Nature's own miracle moisturiser and the mineral water adds a refreshing tingle to get skin stimulated and refine the texture. Leave the mask on for 10 to 15 minutes, then rinse off with tepid mineral water or pure water.

MEADOWSWEET

Meadowsweet (*Filipendula ulmaria*) has traditionally been used for its cleansing properties and its sweet, light scent. It also has a soothing and slightly sedative effect. A simple and pleasurable way of using this herb is in a bath bag. Use five parts meadowsweet to two parts lime flowers to one part pelargonium (scented geranium) leaves. Place the herbs in a muslin or cheesecloth bag and suspend it on a string beneath the hot water tap so that the water runs through it into the tub, thus extracting all the properties from the herbs. Afterwards, rub the bag briskly over the body like a sponge, squeezing the juices from the herbs.

Meadowsweet bathwater may be made by simmering together equal parts of meadowsweet flowers, fine oatmeal and bran in a large pan of water covered with a tightly fitting lid for at least 1 hour. Remove from heat and allow to cool slightly before straining.

Meadowsweet may also be taken internally, either as a tea or a stronger decoction. It is soothing and healing to the gastrointestinal tract and has a pronounced and positive effect on patients suffering from hyperacidity; it is also indicated in managing a fever and for urinary infections. A recommended therapeutic dose is 2 g of the dried flowers and leaves up to three times a day.

MILK

Tip:

Milk helps chapped or roughened hands; each night, soak hands in a bowl of warm milk for 5 to 10 minutes, rinse off and pat dry with a soft towel.

Baths or showers should be lukewarm, rather than hot, because hot water has the effect of dissolving the protective oil film on the skin, allowing moisture to escape. A warm milk bath is a tried-and-true natural remedy for dry parched skin, chapping of the skin and sensitivity to the touch. Add 2 cups of milk (whole milk rather than low-fat here!) to soften the effects of the water without leaving a sticky residue in the tub.

MILK THISTLE

In Europe, the milk thistle (*Silybum marianum*), with its pronounced white veins, was once thought a 'great breeder of milk and a proper diet for wet nurses [breast-feeding women]', according to herbalist Nicolas Culpeper. More recently, exciting pharmacological research has indicated that milk thistle extract can regenerate liver cells and protect them against toxins which result from overuse of alcohol, drug use or just chemical pollution. Taken as a tea, milk thistle has a pronounced and beneficial effect on the gall bladder digestive system, and helps to stimulate bile flow.

MINT

There are dozens of different kinds of refreshing, cooling mint, including apple mint (*Mentha rotundifolia*), peppermint (M. *piperita*) (see p. 127), pennyroyal (M. *pulegium*) (see p. 126) and eau-de-Cologne mint (M. *piperita citrata*). All have been valued for medicinal as well as culinary uses since very early times. Apple mint, for instance, was once known as 'the monk's herb' because monks used it to make jellies which were served to recuperating patients. Spearmint (M. *spicata*) (see p. 151) is probably best known as a kitchen herb; peppermint and pennyroyal are more frequently employed for medicinal purposes.

The Greeks and Romans crowned themselves with mint for banquets and put bunches on the table in the hope of warding off drunkenness. Ending a meal with a sprig of mint to help the digestion and sweeten the breath is a very ancient custom, culminating in the widespread popularity of 'after dinner mints', still used today. Mints were used for scenting bathwater, being thought to 'strengthen the sinewes' at the same time. They were also used as strewing herbs and grown near food crops to keep rats and mice at bay. This is still a good tip — if you are plagued by mice or other vermin, leave rags soaked in peppermint oil near where their nest is. They hate the smell. Similarly, crushed mint was placed in mattresses and linen presses as the smell deterred fleas.

MOTHERWORT

Motherwort or lion's ear (*Leonurus cardiaca*) is a bitter tonic herb, formerly much used to speed delivery in childbirth. Herbalists will prescribe it during the last few weeks of pregnancy for its effect upon the uterus. It may be listed as an ingredient in a women's tonic or nutritional supplement, and is quite safe and beneficial as a female tonic herb and glandular balancer in the small quantities therein. A professional herbalist may prescribe motherwort tea for painful periods, especially where they are associated with nervous tension, and for disturbed menstrual cycles in general. Motherwort is also a natural remedy for cardiovascular-related tension problems, notably for tachycardia and palpitations. However, it should not be taken unless under the guidance of a professional therapist.

MULBERRY

Mulberries (*Morus nigra*) have been grown in Asia and parts of Europe since ancient times. In the past they were grown in Mesopotamia, where seeds of the fruits have been excavated, and they have even been found in early Egyptian tombs. It seems probable that mulberries became popular in these early cultures because of the thirst-quenching properties of their delicious fruit. They were also cultivated as food for silkworms.

The Romans were the first to praise the mulberry both as a food and as a medicine. It is often mentioned in their early writings as a gargle for diseases of the mouth and as a medicine for stomach complaints and digestive disorders. According to the mediaeval Doctrine of Signatures, the appearance of a herb or plant dictated its use as a medicine. Thus, for instance, toothwort, with its whitish scales, was used to treat toothache, while the plum-coloured juice of the mulberry was used to staunch bleeding and for all circulatory disorders. Heresbachius wrote in 1578 that 'Of the Mulberie is made a very noble medicine for the stomacke, and for the Goutes that will longest endure kept in glasses'.

MULLEIN

The yellow flowers of mullein or Aaron's rod (*Verbascum thapsus*) provide an excellent earache oil to relieve pain. Steep the flowers in oil in sunlight for 3 weeks, then strain out the flowers and add fresh ones to the oil. Repeat the process two to three times. Similarly, mullein oil or tea may be used to treat inflammations of the throat and bronchial tubes, for a dry cough or bronchial spasm, or for painful, hard coughing. Mullein oil is also available from your health food store and those pharmacies which specialise in homoeopathic preparations.

MUSTARD

Mustard powder and seeds are excellent rubefacients, meaning they have a warming effect on the skin and flesh and will help to reduce pain. A mustard poultice encourages blood flow towards the surface in cases of rheumatism, sciatica, neuralgia and various internal inflammations, also. To make a mustard plaster, add sufficient tepid water and flour to 1 tablespoon of crushed mustard seeds to make a thick paste. Place the mixture in a folded cloth and apply to the painful area. (Note: if skin is delicate or dry, massage the area with olive oil first and do not leave plaster on for more than 5 minutes. Check at this point, to ensure the skin is not unduly reddened or burned.)

The old-fashioned mustard bath revives cold and wet feet and helps to ward off a chill. Blend 3 tablespoons of mustard powder to a paste with a little water and add to a bowl of hot water, large enough to place both feet in comfortably. Soak feet for 15 minutes.

MYRRH

Hippocrates advised an interesting cure for a toothache or abscess — 'Scratch the gum with the tooth of a man who has suffered a violent death'! This certainly is not very practical, so to cope with the pain, try applying tincture of myrrh (*Commiphora myrrha*). Myrrh is very antiseptic, astringent and healing and will immediately ease mouth sores or fungal infections. Add a few drops of myrrh tincture to sherry for a cleansing (but bitter tasting, be warned!) mouthwash. A gargle made with salt, vinegar and myrrh tincture may be used as an emergency measure for a decayed tooth or cavity while waiting to see a dentist.

NASTURTIUM

Although nasturtiums (*Tropaeolum major*) are not, strictly speaking, available for sale in health food stores and pharmacies, you may well find them listed as an ingredient on the packs of antidandruff preparations or skin care products, tonics or tablets aimed at helping to treat adolescent acne.

Not only are the flowers, leaves and seed pods of the nasturtium all edible and flavoursome, with a subtle peppery taste, but the flowers in particular contain large amounts of vitamin C. This makes them a valuable internal and external treatment for warding off infections. Nasturtiums are also one of 'nature's antibiotics', containing a generous serving of sulphur which is a well-known skin clearer. If you suffer from acne, try making your own skin tonic in the following fashion: chop and steep a dozen leaves for 10 minutes in boiling water, then drink the liquid three times a day. This infusion could be used as a wash or a facial steam, too, for badly troubled skin.

Tip:

To encourage hair growth, mix a few drops of nasturtium essence (from perfumers or essential oil suppliers) with rosemary oil and rub into your scalp.

NETTLE

These plants are ancient in origin. Nettles' (*Urtica dioica*) use in healing dates back to the 3rd century BC when Hippocrates prescribed nettles as a poultice to treat snakebites and scorpion stings. A very old use for nettles is as a vegetable side dish. The young leaves can be cooked and served rather like spinach and the stems may be parboiled and dressed with a sauce to accompany most meat dishes.

Dried nettle tea is rich in iron, making it a useful tonic. Taken with or without lemon and honey,

Tip:

In addition to being a natural remedy, nettles are a useful natural preservative. If you have a glut of soft fruit, tomatoes or root vegetables from your home garden, pack them in dried nettle leaves: this will make them last longer.

it is also a surprisingly tasty one and particularly appropriate for a recuperating patient. As well as being rich in iron, nettles are a good source of large amounts of all the vitamins and minerals, like all 'greedy feeders' that rob the soil of nutrients. In herbal medicine, nettles are used as a circulatory stimulant — in ancient Rome, soldiers would beat their arms and legs with stinging nettles to warm themselves up and they are still to be found listed as an ingredient in rubbing preparations for rheumatism patients and for those with poor peripheral circulation.

Tip:

To condition the scalp, make an infusion of stinging nettle, and apply — this will dilate the blood vessels of the scalp and encourage healthy growth.

In seeming contrast, the crushed fresh leaves may also be infused to create a cooling and healing poultice, suitable for patients with infantile or allergic eczema. Taken either as a tea or as a dose of up to 3 g of the dried powdered herb, nettles can have a diuretic effect, making them useful for gout patients. Nettles may also be used for their cosmetic effect. They have a pronounced astringent and toning ability, and therefore dried nettles and nettle essence are both to be found in certain shampoos, especially antidandruff varieties and other preparations for problem hair.

Tip:

If you would like to put the nettles in your garden to good use, dry the leaves (this gets rid of the sting) and use them throughout the year as a potherb. They add a strong and wholesome flavour to stews and soups, as well as being an excellent source of vitamins and iron.

NUTMEG

Grated nutmeg (*Myristica fragrans*) is an invaluable aid in digestive discomfort, including diarrhoea, nervous dyspepsia, vomiting, intestinal spasm and inflammatory diseases affecting the gut. It may also be used for flatulence. Its actions as an antispasmodic and digestive tonic are due to its high concentration of volatile oils, including pinene and eugenol (also found in cloves). Add a tiny amount of grated fresh nutmeg to a cup of ginger tea. A diluted version of this recipe (2:1, boiled water to spiced tea) is also useful as a natural remedy for dealing with colic.

Tip:

To make a spicy mouthwash, soak 1 teaspoon each of nutmeg, peppercorns and rosemary in 150 ml of apple cider vinegar or red wine for 2 weeks; strain before use. Chopped ginger root may also be included: if so, used warm, this will also soothe swollen tonsils or a sore throat.

OATS

Oats (*Avena sativa*) are a great nerve tonic and stimulant for a sluggish digestive system. They form an important restorative in nervous conditions and exhaustion after illness, and are a tonic for insomnia. However, their primary use must be for their nutritional value. Oats have a very beneficial action on the heart muscle and on the urinary organs. Recent research has pointed to the beneficial effects of including oat bran in the diet, as it has a marked ability to lower cholesterol levels in the body. Oats are of particular benefit in special diets for convalescents and those suffering from gastroenteritis and dyspepsia.

Tip:

Keep a small bowl of raw oat bran near the sink. Dip neglected hands in, rub thoroughly and then rinse to cleanse them. This is much gentler on your hands than soap — remember, your hands, like your lips, do not contain many sebaceous glands, meaning they are very prone to dryness, so every little bit of protection helps.

Oats are high in nutrients essential to skin health, including vitamin A, calcium, and the vitamin B complex. Oatmeal is a gentle cleansing agent and will leave a dry skin feeling silky and smooth. Oatmeal soap, made by the addition of oat straw to commercial soap, has long been a specialty item for the coddling of sensitive skin, or for soothing a baby's nappy rash.

Try making a 'gruel' from natural oats and adding it to your bathwater, along with soothing violet or chamomile flowers and some finely chopped orange peel, to remedy dry, itchy skin, eczema or insect bites.

Honey 'n' Oat Mask

1 *tablespoon sesame, avocado or sunflower oil*

1 *tablespoon raw honey*

1 *dessertspoon rolled oats*

Gently lubricate hands and face with oil. Apply a light film of raw pure honey, thickening it with rolled oats to achieve a mask-like consistency. Lying in the gentle early morning or late afternoon sun for no more than 10 minutes can speed the effects of the treatment. Then rinse off with tepid water and pat dry with a soft towel.

OILS, COLD-PRESSED

The skin's outermost layer should contain about 15 per cent water. When that water content falls below 10 per cent, the skin becomes noticeably dry. The body's own defence against this dryness is the natural oil, sebum, that it produces continually to keep the skin lubricated and soft. However, this has little chance against the onslaught of hot summer winds or cold winter ones, or against any of the sudden changes in temperature in between which often result in dry, parched skin. Over-dry homes or offices, where the humidity is at most 15 per cent, mean that the moisture in the outer layer of your skin is transpired into the atmosphere faster than it can be replaced. This can seriously dehydrate skin and hair. In addition to drinking more water, it is a good idea to take a dessertspoon of pure cold-pressed oil daily to provide a food source for the internal manufacture of sebum. Either take it 'neat' or mix it in with a salad dressing or other recipe.

Tip:

Dry skin requires constant lubrication to prevent flaking and premature ageing. One of the easiest ways to provide this is to put a tablespoon of cold-pressed oil into a daily bath. You might like to try this blend for your bath. Take 200 ml Turkey red oil, 20 ml rose oil and 50 ml avocado oil and mix well in a tightly lidded jar or bottle.

Cold-pressed oils are used in cosmetics as preservatives and also to soften the skin. Wheat germ oil is healing and contains vitamin E, while almond oil is a valuable skin food (but expensive). Castor oil is a strengthening hair oil, and a specially treated castor oil, sometimes called 'Turkey red oil', disperses in water and so can also be used in the bath.

An oil bath will do wonders for your skin. Select from the range of naturally scented cold-pressed oils at your health food store or pharmacy. Add a few tablespoons to warm bathwater — apricot and almond oils are very good, and so are sesame, avocado and olive oils (olive oil is rich and emollient but occasionally strong-smelling).

OLIVE OIL

Olive oil can be used for bowel disorders and as a laxative. Because of its mild action, olive oil can be especially good for young children and pregnant women. It is good for constipation, colic and in cases of diarrhoea which are actually due to faulty digestion (irritable bowel syndrome) rather than to a viral infection. Olive oil is a traditional remedy for expelling worms from the system.

In AD 60, Dioscorides wrote: 'But ye oyle which is of the wild olive is more binding and the second in use for ye state of health. It is convenient instead of Rosaceum for ye Caput dolentibus, stays sweatings, and the haire falling. It doth cleanse Furfures, and ulcera capitas manantia, and scabiem, and Lepras, and it keeps off gray haires a long tyme from them which are anointed therewith dayly.'

Hot olive oil treatments help combat dryness and improve the health of the hair. Part your hair into sections and apply the oil along the parts with a cotton ball. Cover the entire scalp. Then wring out a towel in hot water and wrap it around your head and leave in place until it cools. Repeat the towel treatment seven or eight times. Then wash with a natural shampoo.

If you prefer, you can use the heat from a bonnet-type drier. After applying the olive oil, cover your head and sit under the drier for 45 minutes. Better still, you can leave the oil on overnight. Put a shower cap over your head and sleep that way.

OLIVE OIL AND HONEY HAIR CONDITIONER

¾ cup olive oil (the greener the better)

3 tablespoons honey

2 teaspoons sesame oil

Combine all ingredients in a lidded jar and shake well. Leave in the refrigerator between uses.

OLIVE OIL CREAM

2 tablespoons olive oil

2 tablespoons lanolin

Melt ingredients together in a bowl standing in simmering water. Mix and leave to cool. Store in a clean tightly lidded glass jar in the refrigerator and apply to dry skin as a daily treatment.

ONION

Onion juice, made into a syrup with honey, is beneficial as a cough medicine. Onion juice may also be used for its antibacterial properties as a poultice for dressing grazes or wounds. Roasted or raw onions can also be applied to a sprain in the form of a poultice.

ORANGE BLOSSOM

The gorgeous scent of these flowers (*Citrus aurantium*) is distilled into an essential oil which is one of the most effective antidepressants around. It has been documented as slowing down and calming the mind and it is very useful for people who tend to panic and for those who are prone to hyperventilation or are under a great deal of strain. It has even been used clinically to treat cardiac patients with great success. Add 4 to 6 drops to a warm bath to soothe and comfort the brain and the body.

Aromatherapists use orange blossom (neroli) oil to

treat patients suffering from anxiety and insomnia because of its sedative properties. They also use it to treat broken veins and dry skin.

It is particularly indicated for use in a facial steam or massage by people with dry, ageing or unduly fragile skin, particularly at the time of menopause.

Orange blossom oil regularly appears as an ingredient in all manner of cosmetics and body care preparations and as a base ingredient of many perfumes.

ORANGE PEEL

A dye to restore colour to grey hair may be made by adding ½ cup vodka to ½ cup of dried, chopped orange peel; allow the mixture to steep in a covered bowl or non-aluminium saucepan for approximately 7 to 10 days. Strain, and discard the peel. Add the mixture to 1 cup peanut oil. Store in a lidded glass jar in the refrigerator, shaking thoroughly before each use.

ORRIS ROOT

Powdered orris root (*Iris florentina*) was used as a sweet-scented hair powder in the 18th century. Today, it is most commonly used as a fixative in potpourri and sachet mixes.

However, in cases of illness, or another occasion when you are unable to wash your hair, try a dry shampoo with finely ground orris root. Gently pat the orris root powder through the hair: it will remove grease from the hair by absorption. Brush in, then brush through thoroughly.

PANTHENOL

If you are plagued by split ends or a thicket of dull lack-lustre hair, panthenol can give more results than most forms of protein. In tests conducted in Europe and the USA, it has been scientifically proven that this provita-min form of B_5 actually mends split ends and attracts moisture into the inner core of the hair's structure. One catch though: for panthenol to work, it must be used every few days and needs to stay on your hair for between 10 and 20 minutes. This means you should select a conditioner or deep conditioning treatment con-taining this ingredient for best results; a shampoo, which is washed out within a minute or so, is less likely to be of benefit.

PARA-AMINOBENZOIC ACID

Para-aminobenzoic acid or PABA has been shown to help prevent greying hair and to maintain healthy skin and hair. Food sources are brewer's yeast, wholegrain products, dairy foods, wheat germ, fresh fruit and green vegetables. Some results of deficiency include poor skin and hair growth, loss of hair, fatigue and some forms of eczema.

PARSLEY

Parsley (*Petroselinum crispum*) has been widely grown and used for thousands of years, both as a garnish and flavouring and as a medicinal tonic herb. Being one of the first plants to appear in spring, it has been used in the Jewish Passover meal of Seder to symbolise a new start. The Greeks esteemed it as a healthful herb, and when someone was ill they described them as 'being in need of parsley'. Homer wrote that warriors fed their chariot horses with parsley before combat and that victorious athletes were crowned with parsley chaplets. The Romans wore necklaces of parsley and scattered sprigs all along their banqueting tables, believing this prevented drunkenness. The seeds were once eaten by both men and women in the mistaken belief that this encouraged fertility.

Parsley is almost as rich in vitamin A as cod liver oil. It is also rich in iron, making it a useful supplement for anyone suffering from anaemia. It is rich in vitamin C, calcium and other minerals. Parsley should be used liberally in food served to a recuperating patient for it stimulates the entire digestive system, thus 'perking up' the appetite. As long ago as 1597, John Gerard wrote that 'Parsley be also delightful to the taste, and agreeable to the stomacke'. Parsley has long been highly regarded as a kidney tonic and, indeed, it does have a strong diuretic effect, thus helping to flush out any infection or toxins in the system. For this reason, parsley tea was routinely served to troops during World War I to cure kidney problems which often accompanied dysentery.

Tip:
Parsley contains one of the highest levels of chlorophyll of any herb, making it a very effective breath freshener.

The crushed wetted leaves make a soothing dressing for bruises, insect bites or minor grazes, as well as being a remedy for rheumatism. Taken internally, and applied externally as a skin tonic lotion, parsley is thought to help clear reddened or itchy skin and pimples. Parsley simmered in wine was an old wives' remedy for sore breasts in new mothers. Parsley infused in oil was used to bind sprains and a wad of cotton wool soaked in cooled parsley tea was a remedy for toothache. Interesting new research indicates that, due to its apparent antihistamine action, parsley may help those susceptible to hay fever or hives.

Try this invigorating recipe.

PARSLEY SCRUB

2 tablespoons fresh parsley, chopped
50 g almond meal
50 g fuller's earth
150 ml water

Infuse the parsley in boiling water for half an hour. Cool, strain and mix parsley liquid with almond meal and fuller's earth to form a paste. Apply the mixture to damp skin with light, circular movements. Rinse skin thoroughly and pat dry with a soft towel.

PAWPAW

Also known as papaya (*Carica papaya*), this fruit has incredible digestive properties, and it is therefore very suitable for all digestive disorders.

PENNYROYAL

Also known as 'pudding grass' and *organie*, pennyroyal (*Mentha pulegium*) is a pungent low-growing herb, with circlets of mauve flowers in spring. With its small smooth leaves and its fresh sweet smell, it makes a delightful ground cover. Pennyroyal has been held in great esteem for its ability to repel fleas. It is a very good idea to dab pennyroyal oil in your dog's kennel so he is not troubled by these pests. Similarly, either the neat oil or a diluted version can be rubbed on the skin as protection against mosquitoes, dabbed on shelving to repel moths from clothing or used in the pantry against ants.

Sailors used to purify their drinking water with pennyroyal. You might like to try an infusion for coughs, hoarseness and indigestion, or use daily as a refreshing mouthwash. Pennyroyal oil is sometimes included in natural fluoride-free toothpastes. The herb is occasionally available as a prepared tea or in tea bags. (Note: pennyroyal oil and tea should not be taken during pregnancy.) Pennyroyal has also been used cosmetically — Nicolas Culpeper recommended a mashed paste of leaves to soothe rashes and treat pimples and inflammation.

Make your own pennyroyal insect repellent. Take 200 ml olive or apricot kernel oil and place in a non-aluminium saucepan. Cook until the oil is well heated, then stir in a heaped teaspoon of dried pennyroyal. Simmer over low heat for 35 to 40 minutes. Then filter out the herb and bottle the oil. To use, apply to exposed skin. It is a nourishing skin treat too!

PEPPERMINT

Peppermint (*Mentha piperita*) is extremely useful as a digestive herb. English herbalist Nicolas Culpeper wrote 'Mint is very profitable to the stomach, especially to dissolve wind and help the colic'. In Roman times, the leaves were rubbed over banquet tables to 'stir up a greedy taste for meate'. Pregnant women experiencing nausea may find great relief with a cup of peppermint tea: this is mentioned in both old and new herbals as a natural remedy for morning sickness. (Note: Only a standard mild peppermint tea infusion should be taken as a too-strong one can prove dangerous when pregnant.)

Tip:

Herbalists will often prescribe peppermint tea for a patient who has difficulty digesting milk products. It is a useful digestive tonic and will have a pronounced effect on the appetite.

Greek and Roman physicians prescribed peppermint for just about everything, from hiccups to leprosy. A very old remedy for a bee or wasp sting is to rub it with mint leaves. In more recent times, chemists distilled menthol from peppermint oil and this is used in a wide variety of medicines, especially those which you might be prescribed to help prevent stomach ulcers and stimulate bile secretion. Menthol also appears in various products to relieve congestion, such as Vicks Vaporub. Peppermint and peppermint essence were also important ingredients in early tooth-cleaning preparations and remain so today.

A mild washing water made from peppermint leaves is a cooling face lotion for those with sensitive skin. Traditionally, peppermint has been used as a steam-cleansing herbal treatment for the face. Add 2 tablespoons of the leaves to boiling water in a large bowl or sink. Hold your face close to the steam and drape a towel over your head and the bowl rim. After steaming your face for 15 minutes, wipe with dampened cotton wool to remove impurities, then close the pores by splashing with cold water. For a total facial treatment, apply a face mask and then tone with a minty infusion.

> **Tip:**
> Drinking peppermint tea will help overcome sore muscles and cramps. You can apply it externally as a wet mash to the area also, as its camphoraceous principles will help to relieve pain.

> **Tip:**
> If you grow peppermint, you can easily make your own peppermint oil by macerating the fresh leaves in a fine carrier oil — apricot kernel or almond oil, preferably — for up to 2 months. Strain before use.

PERILLA

Perilla (*Perilla frutescens*) is also known as beefsteak plant, and *shiso* in Japan, and you may come across it in health food stores and Japanese specialty food shops, especially those which supply herbs and spices. Perilla has been used as a natural remedy to counter food poisoning, presumably for its powerful tonic effect on the digestive system. Pickled plums or *umeboshi*, which contain perilla, are a popular means of countering colic and flatulence in Asian countries. The salted leaves, which are also available pre-packed in some Asian stores, may be eaten as an appetiser for the same reason.

PHOSPHORUS

Exhausted? It might be the result of prolonged exposure to the sun, to nervous stress, or simply too much exercise. However, even if you are in good condition, it is easy to misjudge your reserves. A phosphorus deficiency may be indicated by loss of appetite, fatigue, nervous disorders, weight loss, nervous eczema or inflamed and itchy skin that has flared up for no apparent reason. Almonds, beans, lentils and whole-wheat foods are the highest vegetable sources of phosphorus. Other food sources include eggs, fish, glandular meats and poultry. Phosphorus tablets, capsules and compounds are available but it's important to eat well and regularly. Excess dieting can make you feel weak and wrung out. Start the day with homemade sugar-free muesli and an egg any which way.

Phosphorus is also the 'bone builder', helping to build healthy bones, teeth and hair. It also plays an important role in the body's metabolising of fats and carbohydrates.

PINE

Essential oil of pine (*Picea abies*) is listed as an ingredient in various warming rubs and liniments. It is a stimulating herbal essence and naturally antiseptic. Use it in a bath for its fragrant and toning effects, and for its ability to relax sore muscles; it is also a fine air freshener.

PLANTAIN

Plantain (*Plantago major*) has bactericidal properties and crushed, heated plantain leaves have been used since very early times to draw and heal abscesses and boils. Even city dwellers can find plantain in parks. This plant has exceptional styptic properties, meaning it is strongly astringent and cleansing. Make a tea of the whole plant and use this infusion as a dressing, either directly on a wound or added to a warm bath for a long, soothing soak.

Plantain tincture and salve are easily made and are a must for anybody's medicine cabinet. To prepare the tincture, soak a handful of the leaves in enough brandy to cover and store in a warm place for 2 weeks. Strain and mix with distilled water. The salve may be made by combining 2 teaspoons of plantain juice — made by pulping and sieving the leaves — with 150 g pure white lard. Melt together over low heat, strain and store in the refrigerator in a clean glass jar.

POPPY

Poppy (*Papaver rhoeas*) petals are probably best known for the splash of colour they add to a garden. However, did you know they may be used as a surprisingly effective natural aid in the war against wrinkles? Take one handful of the petals — don't worry about which colour — and infuse them in 250 ml boiling water; allow to steep for 10 to 15 minutes. Strain the liquid and allow to cool before using as a skin tonic or, diluted with distilled water, as a facial 'mist' when applying make-up. This blend will keep refrigerated for up to 2 weeks.

POTASSIUM

This mineral is valuable to take as a supplement during recuperation; it also helps counter constipation, especially in an elderly housebound patient. Good food sources include dates, figs, peaches, tomatoes, blackstrap molasses, peanuts, raisins and seafood. Some symptoms of deficiency include acne, dry skin, insomnia, nervousness, nervous eczema, greasy skin and sudden hair loss.

POTATO

Potatoes (*Solanum tuberosum*) are the richest natural source of potassium chloride, and raw potatoes can be very useful in first aid. Use a raw, peeled, grated potato around a sprain of any kind. Hot baked potato pulp can also be applied to relieve tennis elbow or other joint pain. If you are in a great deal of pain, for instance after having a wisdom tooth out, try a hot potato poultice. Spread slices of boiled, peeled potatoes between pieces of flannel and apply to your cheek, as hot as can be tolerated.

Tip:

Chapped hands are sore and inconvenient. One of the oddest-sounding and most effective remedies for this condition is leftover cooked mashed potato, mixed with a little almond oil and orange flower water.

POWDERS

Body powders are cooling, smoothing and fragrant — a delightful addition to a bath experience.

Tip:

Did you know a potato is a simple and effective skin freshener? Simply rub the skin with a chilled slice of raw potato; it will help to close the pores and refine the texture of the skin.

Loosely fill a china jar with the bruised petals of fragrant flowers picked at the height of their scent. Gardenia, jasmine and rose all have a strong scent which is distinctive yet delicate. Add cornstarch or arrowroot and a teaspoon of rice. Cover. After 2 weeks, sift the mixture into a jar with a secure lid and add a powder puff. An excellent cooling and absorbent baby powder is made by combining two parts of arrowroot, one part chamomile flowers and one part calendula flowers, and grinding them to a fine powder.

PSYLLIUM

For constipation, always start with the mildest cure, which is a diet including prunes, apples, spinach and figs. Failing that, try psyllium (*Plantago psyllium*) powder or granules. Put 1 tablespoon in a 300 ml glass of warm water and leave until it has developed into a gelatinous mass, then drink it. It has the appearance of frog spawn, but do persevere. It is quite tasteless and very effective. Several cereal companies are now including psyllium fibre in their breakfast products, for it has also been shown to be advantageous to a heart-healthy diet.

PURSLANE

Purslane (*Portulaca oleracea*) is a valuable little herb with cooling, tonic and aperient effects. It is sometimes listed as an ingredient in various slimming preparations and metabolic tonics. It is rich in vitamins and minerals, making it a valuable 'skin and hair' food supplement. It is easily grown and quite palatable, so you might like to get into the habit of using a few of the fresh leaves in a salad; alternatively, you may dry the leaves and use them to make a tea. Add 1 teaspoon of the dried herb to 1 cup of boiling water, strain and drink.

QUINCE

An excellent naturally based hair-setting lotion can be derived from the quince (*Cydonia oblonga*). Measure 50 g of quince seed and boil in 275 ml of water for 15 minutes. Make up the quantity of liquid, if necessary, as it evaporates. Strain the mixture and press through muslin, making sure that as much mucilage as possible is squeezed through. The liquid will jellify and set when cold. Apply either hot or warm, as preferred.

RASPBERRY

That raspberries belong to the rose (*Rosaceae*) family should come as no surprise to those who have picked them and snagged clothing or scratched fingers on the prickly canes in the attempt.

The raspberry was much admired as a medicine by the Greeks and Romans. Pliny the Elder noted 'A third kind the Greeks called the Ida bramble . . . its blossom is used to make an ointment for sore eyes, and also, dipped in honey, for St Anthony's Fire [erysipelas] and also, soaked in water, it makes a draught to cure stomach troubles'. By the 17th century, medical and household writers were both making enthusiastic mention of raspberries. Worlidge, in 1697, said raspberries ought not to be omitted from any garden, as they 'yield one of the most pleasant juices of any fruit and make an excellent wine, invaluable for mothers and their babes'.

Herbalists still prescribe a tea made from raspberry leaves to assist mothers during childbirth. Raspberry leaf tablets and capsules are sold in pharmacies and health food stores and are claimed to speed delivery and help the uterus to contract after labour. (Note: As with all medications to be taken during pregnancy, it is strongly recommended that any herbal preparations, including this one, are only taken under the supervision of a qualified medical practitioner or herbalist.) Severe pelvic pain may be temporarily treated with a compound containing herbs, such as raspberry leaf, specifically indicated for their regulatory effect on the gynaecological system. However, pain is an obvious indication that all is not well, so see your doctor promptly.

The berries themselves are a good source of vitamins A and C, calcium, phosphorus, iron, potassium and thiamine. Raspberry 'shrub' is a traditional drink made by steeping the berries in wine or cider vinegar and is said to help relieve a fever and to calm a fractious child. It is also thought to have a beneficial regulatory effect on the heart.

RED CLOVER

The sweet-smelling, honey-tasting flower heads of red clover (*Trifolium pratense*) may be gathered fresh and brewed into a delicious and nerve-soothing tea; red clover tea and tea bags are also available and make a viable alternative if you are endeavouring to find a beverage more soothing to the nerves than coffee or regular tea. Red clover tea helps promote sleep; an infusion may also be used to cleanse and dress minor wounds, having very mild antiseptic properties. Red clover essence is sometimes used as an ingredient in hair or bath preparations, by virtue of its delectable scent.

REDCURRANT

By the 15th century, redcurrants (*Ribes rubrum*) were being cultivated as a border plant and as a food source. Redcurrants were much used for flavouring meat and fish dishes; they were also thought to have certain medicinal properties. The 16th century herbalist William Turner wrote in 1568 'The juyce and syrope of Ribes are good for hote agues and agaynst hote fires and vomitings of choler . . . They provoke appetite and quenche thyrste.' Redcurrants do contain a fair amount of vitamin C (although not as much as blackcurrants), which makes them very useful for patients with fever. They are also an excellent source of vitamin A, iron and thiamine, some phosphorus, calcium, riboflavin, niacin and potassium.

ROSE

Essential oil of rose is soothing and antiseptic; aroma-therapists use it as a sedative and antidepressant tonic for patients. It may be used as a soother for sensitive skin, nervous tension and menstrual cramps. It is also indicated for use as a remedy in the treatment of acne, eczema, herpes and ulcers. Make a massage oil by adding rose essence or oil to almond or olive oil. Bathrooms, toilets and baby's nursery can be made to smell sweet by cotton balls perfumed with rose oil tucked under change tables or behind cisterns. Add 1 or 2 drops to a sponge and rub the skirting boards of your home to create a sweet-smelling and relaxing atmosphere.

Tip:

Add 2 to 3 drops of ros[e] essence to the exhaus[t] of your vacuum cleane[r] and the fragrance wil[l] spread.

ROSEHIPS

Rosehips are the fruit of the rose. Rosehip tea, rosehip syrup and rosehip tablets may be taken for their tonic effect on the system, rosehips being an excellent and potent natural source of vitamin C. This is also the traditional herb for treating dilated capillaries, those small, red, broken lines which give the skin a somewhat weathered look. Rosehip tea is a delicious and effective 'skin drink'; cooled, the tea may also be used on a compress for reddened or strained eyes.

Rosehips are also high in bioflavonoids, which contribute to the quality of collagen tissues. The tissues supporting the top layers of skin are made up of collagen, the fibrous support which, when plump, keeps skin looking youthful. But when it sags and thins down, it contributes to a wrinkled look of premature ageing (think of what a sagging bedspring does to a mattress!) Many expensive cosmetic products contain collagen, usually derived from animal slaughter by-products, but it is far better to maintain your skin's elastic condition from within with a good health diet. In Sweden, rosehips are a popular health food to which experts such as Dr Paavo

Airola have attributed the naturally beautiful skin of Swedish women.

ROSEMARY

Rosemary (*Rosmarinus officinalis*) has been recorded in every herbal and medical text since very early times, and it has long been regarded as a preserver of youth. Even just smelling rosemary was thought 'to keep thee youngly'. It was mentioned in one of the earliest English herbals, *The Leech Book of Bald*, as a skin tonic, with instructions to 'boyle the leves in whyte wine and wasshe thy face therewith . . . thou shall have a fayre face . . . wash thyself and thou shalt waxe shiny'. From then on, rosemary was one of the most popular of herbs, admired and used for its many medicinal, culinary and aromatic uses.

Tip:

With its refreshing natural perfume, rosemary is useful when making potpourri and toilet waters. Lay rosemary amongst woollens as a moth deterrent.

Bunches of rosemary were burned during times of plague in a bid to ward off infection, and judges and jury members held sprigs of rosemary when attending the courtroom to dispel any 'jail fever' the criminal may have brought along. The French hung rosemary in hospitals as a kind of healing incense and rosemary leaves were burned in field hospitals as recently as World War II for their antiseptic and purifying effect on the air. By the same token, you might like to burn rosemary oil in an incense burner in a sick room; this is particularly useful for patients suffering from respiratory complaints, such as colds and flu, as it helps to clear the sinuses and head.

Rosemary has been much researched and used as a medicinal herb. It was first noted as having preservative qualities centuries ago when meat was wrapped in crushed rosemary leaves to stop it from spoiling. By association, rosemary was used in many preparations to restore youth, care for the skin and retard wrinkles, cure paralysis and ease the aches and pains of diseases associated with ageing.

A tea made from fresh rosemary is beneficial for headaches, and like most herbs which have a time-honoured culinary application, it is also an excellent digestive aid. With its powerful aroma, a distillation of rosemary oil is an effective inhalant and decongestant. Rub oil of rosemary on a child's chest to ease a cough. You will note that several antispasmodic chest rubs contain rosemary oil, possibly along with other decongestant herbs and essences such as oil of wintergreen and camphor.

Rosemary oil is a common ingredient in many preparations and massage rubs for painful arthritic joints. Rosemary tea or water is a tasty and effective gargle to treat bad breath, especially if it is combined with a sweeter herb, such as lemon balm, for daily use.

Rosemary oil has a pleasant aroma because it contains volatile oils similar to camphor that give it a sharp, pine-like scent. Add rosemary tea or oil to bathwater to improve circulation, and use rosemary-based ointment to deal with mild cases of eczema. Rosemary oil is an excellent rinse for oily hair and skin. Rosemary extracts are commonly found in commercial hair rinses and will remove excessive oil secretions and promote thicker hair.

Tip:
A strong tea, made from one part rosemary to approximately five parts boiling water, will also help to relieve a bruise.

Cures for baldness have been sought throughout history. Contemporary herbalists recommend scalp massage with rosemary oil or tea to prevent premature baldness. Make a strong infusion from rosemary — or the oil — and rub into the scalp three or four times each week. An old gipsy remedy for greying hair calls for a very strong brew of rosemary: this has a proven stimulating effect on the circulation of the scalp and also helps to get rid of dandruff and stimulate hair growth.

ROSEWATER

Rosewater is a traditional and safe natural cosmetic which can be used as a soothing lotion or compress for sore or inflamed skin. Wipe diluted rosewater (2:1, purified water to rosewater) over the eyes with a clean cosmetic sponge to refresh and tone. For compresses, soak a piece of clean lint or cotton in pure rosewater and lay over eyes, throat, cheeks and chin for 10 minutes whilst lying down. Rosewater is also a simple and surprisingly effective treatment for inflamed or burned skin. Combine it, half and half, with witch hazel for an economical and effective skin toner or all-over body splash.

You might like to try making your own rosewater with the produce of your garden — the only cost is a little time, enjoyably invested in your own pleasure. An infusion of red rose petals may be easily prepared by placing a handful of the flowers in boiling water and simmering for 10–15 minutes. Strain, then cool before use.

RUE

Rue (*Ruta graveolens*) was once known as the herb of grace, by association with 'rue' meaning repentance. The leaves may be crushed to make a very refreshing if somewhat pungent tea. Rue also has a long history of medicinal use and Milton mentioned its use for eye ailments. Along with lavender, rue was a chief constituent of the famed 'Four Thieves Vinegar', said to have been used by robbers during the Great Plague of Marseilles; they washed their hands and faces with the powerfully scented vinegar before stealing from the homes of ill people and never caught the disease themselves. The 9th century monk Wilfrid Strabo noted that 'great is its powre over evil odours' and Nicholas Culpeper wrote in the 17th century that the leaves were used to strew the floors of prisons and workhouses to reduce the risk of infection.

SAGE

Sage (*Salvia officinalis*) is an ancient herb, having been held in high repute as a culinary and medicinal plant since Classical times. It is interesting that the generic name, *salvia*, comes from Latin words for health and it has a very broad medicinal reputation.

A Greek physician wrote of it as 'Sage the Saviour', and recommended it be used to ease headaches and nervous tension, to promote menstruation and as a remedy for almost all kidney complaints. Sage was at one time thought to confer longevity, with John Evelyn writing that 'In short, 'tis a plant endow'd with so many and wonderful properties that the assiduous use of it is said to render men immortal'.

> **Tip:**
> Sage is a useful first aid herb around the house. For cuts and scrapes, crush a sage leaf and apply it to the wound before washing and bandaging it.

Sage tea is a refreshing tonic drink and has been considered an important medicinal beverage for several thousand years. An old saying goes 'How can a man die who has sage in his garden?' This is a reference to its use in numerous prescriptions for all known maladies. Sage has an astringent and cooling effect, so may be taken as a spring tonic, a blood cleanser and to promote the appetite. It will also help to cool a fever and ease headaches. Interesting new research points to sage's prowess as a natural deodorant and antiperspirant, with studies showing that sage-based preparations cut perspiration by as much as 30 per cent.

A strong brew of sage tea may be used as a gargle and a mouthwash. You can also rub sage leaves on teeth to whiten them and on gums to strengthen them if they are bleeding. Sage tea was once widely used as a remedy for ague, a malarial fever, and to help ease rheumatism and nervous

> **Tip:**
> For a brilliant polish after cleaning your teeth, rub them with a fresh sage leaf.

and muscular tension or pain. Sage oil may be burned in a sick room to help cleanse and purify the air. A strong infusion of sage may be used regularly to rinse through the hair, to make grey hair seem darker. Or try this recipe which is said to counteract grey hair. Simmer 2 tablespoons of sage in 1 cup of water for 30 minutes, then cover and allow to steep for up to 3 hours. Strain and add 2 tablespoons of rum. Rub it into the hair at the roots two to three times each week. Store in a lidded glass container in the refrigerator, shaking well before each use.

Tip:

A marvellously aromatic honey may be made by steeping a few sage leaves in pure, natural honey. As a bonus, this honey will have added digestive properties.

ST JOHN'S WORT

This pretty perennial (*Hypericum perforatum*) is said to have been named for St John the Baptist. The name is derived from the Greek, meaning 'over an apparition', a reference to its use in mystic rites when it was used to repel evil spirits. St John's wort was also used widely for its medicinal action, being a potent nerve tonic, astringent and expectorant. A tea made from the leaves (25 g of the leaves to 200 ml of water) is useful as a nerve tonic and for catarrh and other lung disturbances. This infusion has also been found effective in countering bedwetting in children.

John Gerard described 'oyle of Saint Jon', made by infusing the herb in olive oil, which would help cleanse wounds 'made by a venom'd weapon'. St John's wort oil is available both by itself or, more often, as an ingredient in another healing cream.

SALAD BURNET

Salad burnet (*Poterium sanguisorba*) has a pleasing cucumber-like flavour and the herb was much used for culinary and medicinal purposes, during mediaeval times in particular. The Hungarians call salad burnet *chabairje*, meaning 'Chaba's salve'. They believe the plant's healing virtues were discovered by King Chaba, who is said to have cured the wounds of 15,000 of his soldiers with it. It was also recommended by herbalist John Gerard 'to make the hart merrie and glad, as also being put into wine, to which it yieldeth a certain grace in drynkynge'.

In early times, it was much used as a salad herb and also in cooling drinks, particularly tankards of cider and wine cups. Try adding a few chopped leaves to iced tea or fresh fruit drinks, especially with fresh strawberry juice (available in health food stores) and watermelon juice. As well as being very tasty, this herb is particularly appropriate for use in dishes and drinks to be served during the hot summer months. It has diaphoretic properties, meaning it encourages light perspiration, thus cooling the skin and reducing overall body temperature.

Salad burnet's Latin name is derived from *sanguis*, meaning blood, and refers to this herb's ability to stem the flow of blood from a cut or other wound. Pliny the Elder recommended a mixture of burnet and honey for treating bruises, boils and abscesses and, along with various other fresh-smelling summer herbs, it was thought to ward off the plague and noxious 'ill humours' which were prevalent during the hotter months. A poultice of the pulped leaves may be used to treat skin problems, such as sunburn or eczema, and a tea made by steeping the leaves may be drunk as a tonic. Salad burnet was once credited with curing gout and rheumatism, although there is no proof for this.

SAVORY

There are two main types of this aromatic plant: the annual summer savory (*Satureja hortensis*) and the perennial winter savory (*Satureja montana*). The delicious-tasting leaves of the bushy annual have long been valued for their flavour and aroma; it was once a traditional strewing herb and may be used in potpourri or posies to good effect. Virgil recommended that summer savory be planted close to beehives. Not only do the inhabitants dote on the nectar-rich flowers, but the pain of a bee or wasp sting is rapidly relieved by rubbing it with crushed summer savory leaves.

'Savory honey', sometimes to be found in health food stores or specialty food shops, is worth seeking out for its very pleasant flavour. Shakespeare mentioned savory in Perdita's bouquet in *The Winter's Tale*, saying that, along with 'hot lavender' and mints, savory should be given to men of middle age. This is a reference to its supposed efficacy as an aphrodisiac. In fact, Richard Banckes in his herbal of 1525 went so far as to say 'It is forbidden to use it much in meates . . . since it stirreth up him that useth it to lechery'.

Savory has a hot spicy 'bite' and was much used in early cookery before pepper became generally affordable. It is traditionally known as the 'bean herb', being used to flavour green beans, broad beans and all sorts of soups or stews based on split or dried beans. As is the case with so many of the culinary herbs which have also served as medicines through the ages, there is a very good reason for this. Not only do the two complement each other in taste, but also beans are notoriously difficult to digest and savory has a tonic and stimulating effect on the digestion. Savory has been recently proved in more modern research to contain certain chemicals that soothe the digestive tract, making it valuable not only as a digestive herb for adults but as a safe adjunct for treating many childhood ailments including colic. The leaves may be brewed as a tea which is soothing to the stomach and quieting to the nerves. It may also be used as a soothing and calming bath herb.

Seventeenth century herbalist Nicolas Culpeper wrote that 'It expels wind from the stomach and bowels . . . Neither is there a better remedy for the colic and iliac passion [upset stomach].' It also had an early reputation as a cough remedy and often appears as an ingredient in natural cough syrups. Another very old use for savory is as a treatment for earache — 'to alleviate singing noises and deafness', Gerard tells us — and for runny eyes.

SEA SALT

This is a boon for dry or cracked skin on the feet. First, to soften the skin, pour 1 cup of sea salt onto a small area in an empty bathtub. Wet it slightly. Sit on the edge of the tub and work your feet back and forth in the salt mixture. Then with your hands, massage the sea salt into your feet, making sure to get all the dry rough areas — sides and tops, too. Rinse with cool water and dry briskly with a towel, rubbing off the old dry skin.

Another salty tonic for tired feet is to prepare two footbaths, one containing hot water to which 1 cup of sea salt has been added, the other with cold water containing an infusion of rosemary. Put feet in the hot water for 5 minutes, then in the cold for 1 minute, back to the hot for 5, back to the cold for 1, and so on. The minerals in the sea salt help to revive and thoroughly clean the skin.

Or try this herb and salt footbath. Take a large handful of fresh sage, thyme or lavender and put in a large bowl with 1 tablespoon of sea salt; cover with boiling water and allow to cool until tolerable.

A very simple and effective tooth powder can also be made with sea salt. Mix 4 teaspoons of ground powdered sage with an equal amount of sea salt and 1 teaspoon of myrrh. Spread the mixture on a baking sheet and place in a slow oven for approximately 30 minutes. Remove and allow to cool slightly, then grind either in a food processor or with a mortar and pestle. Press the mixture through a fine sieve and store in a tightly lidded container. This is a gently abrasive and effectively antibacterial recipe.

SELENIUM

Selenium is an essential mineral which is associated with cancer prevention and a strengthened immune system. It activates the production of coenzyme Q, which in turn stimulates the immune system. In one study, mice treated with coenzyme Q showed significant immune improvement. Researchers at Colorado State University stimulated antibody production in mice up to 30-fold by feeding them selenium. This has enormous implications for the use of this nutrient in preventing diseases. Other studies have used selenium to improve immunity in sheep, dogs and guinea pigs. The nutrient also enhances the effects of certain vaccines, such as the one for malaria.

Selenium deficiency causes a reduction in lymphocytes and phagocytes, the types of immune cells which consume foreign pathogens as they enter the body. As a powerful antioxidant, selenium protects cells throughout the body from damage by free radicals and toxins. This may bestow three related benefits. First, it might diminish the constant level of immune response necessary to deal with free radical damage. Second, it might reduce the auto-immune damage associated with ageing. Third, immune cells may themselves be protected from free radical damage.

At one time scientists thought that selenium had no beneficial role in human nutrition and was itself a potential carcinogen. Now it is very clear that selenium has several important roles in the body and is actually a powerful anticarcinogen and immunostimulant. Selenium supplements can be very useful and safe when

taken wisely, preferably under the supervision of a clinical nutritionist. Soil levels of this mineral (and, therefore, food levels) vary widely, so it is a good idea to
investigate the soil content in your area. Your public
library should be able to help you obtain further details.

SESAME OIL

Sesame (*Sesamum indicum*) oil is a rich fine-textured oil,
which has many cosmetic applications as well as culinary
ones. For instance, a very simple and economical method
for cleaning hands of ingrained dirt is to massage them
thoroughly with a gentle scrub made from equal parts of
raw sugar, sesame oil and lemon juice. A paste made by
adding sesame oil to sea salt is also very good for cleaning rough and grimy skin on knees or elbows.

Sesame oil is about the best natural protection there is
when it comes to sunscreens and is used as the basis of
many commercial preparations. A very old recipe for a
tanning lotion is to combine equal parts of sesame oil
and strong, cold tea, mixing in a bit of lanolin to thicken
the mixture over a slow heat. However, this lotion does
not have enough of the protective qualities that we now
know to be essential for the prevention of premature
wrinkling, dryness and skin cancer and should not be
used as a sunscreen. It does, however, make an excellent
fake bronzing lotion.

SILICA

Silica is the most important mineral for all connective
tissue, skin, hair and nails. Good food sources include
lettuce, strawberries, cucumber, sunflower seeds and
dandelion. Some symptoms of early deficiency can
include poor muscle tone, a change in skin, hair or nail
texture and arthritic nodule formation.

SOAPWORT

Pure herbal shampoos of the past relied on certain plants which contained soapy substances called saponins. One of the best sources of these substances is a perennial bush called 'country soap' or soapwort (*Saponaria officinalis*). For centuries before the advent of commercial soap, this plant was used for all washing purposes and, at one time, it was particularly recommended for washing delicate silks because it gave them a pretty sheen. It is now often listed as an ingredient in natural hair shampoos and cleansing treatments.

Although many good-quality brands of herbal hair care products can now be bought, it is very enjoyable to make your own. Herbal shampoos are made quite easily by pouring boiling water over fresh or dried herbs, leaving them to steep for 24 hours and then straining off the liquid. The usual measure is about 1 heaped teaspoon of herbs — or more if using fresh herbs — to 1 cup of water, but a slightly stronger brew will do no harm at all. If you are using fresh herbs, which are always preferable if available, bruise the leaves before making the infusion to allow the essence to mingle with the water. Add your infusion to a mild organic shampoo or dissolved unscented soap such as Castile soap.

It is possible to procure soapwort root, in either grated or powdered form, from specialist health food stores or via natural products suppliers and distributors — or simply grow it yourself. Make your own shampoo from soapwort root by combining 2 tablespoons of grated or powdered soapwort root with 300 ml of boiling water, mixing and allowing to cool. About ½ cup is needed for a shampoo. Those with greasy hair will find this very effective. When making soapwort shampoo, avoid using metal containers as these can mar the end product. Use china or glazed pottery vessels and stir with a wooden spoon.

SOLOMON'S SEAL

The crushed root of Solomon's seal (*Polygonatum multiflorum*) may be used as a poultice to take away black and blue marks and to help with bruises around the eye. If beer is available, steep the peeled, crushed root in beer and apply on a clean compress to the bruise. To make a soothing rub that will reduce swelling, crush a 5 cm piece of the root and mix with 250 ml wheat germ oil; strain before use. Alternatively, the root may be used to make a strong tea which may be cooled and used as a dressing or wash to help with inflammations, wounds, painful haemorrhoids, allergic reactions to plants and other skin problems. A tea made from the root can also be taken internally for diarrhoea and gastric upsets.

SORREL

There are two main types of sorrel which appear from early summer onwards, one being garden sorrel (*Rumex acetosa*) and the other being French sorrel (R. *scutatus*). The latter is considered the more tasty and succulent but is not necessarily as readily available as garden sorrel. The Romans used it as a condiment to accompany meat, the sharp somewhat citrusy flavour probably helping to break down the effect of fatty, rich meats and game. The use of sorrel reached its peak during Tudor times, when it was widely used as a potherb as well as a medicine, and as a 'salading' in all manner of vegetable dishes and 'pottages'. Although it fell from favour, it is now regaining popularity.

In 1861, Mrs Beeton wrote that 'We gather from the pages of Pliny and Apicius, that sorrel was cultivated by the Romans in order to give them more strength'. Indeed, sorrel is particularly rich in vitamin C, and the leaves were chewed in an effort to avoid scurvy. Sorrel tea and sorrel soup have a cleansing and cooling effect on the system, making them useful for patients recuperating from bladder or kidney ailments. A poultice of warm wetted sorrel leaves will help soothe skin problems and heal minor wounds, the vitamin C content no doubt having a mildly astringent and tonic effect.

Note: Be sparing with sorrel. It is one of the few natural remedies which can have ill effects when taken in large quantities because it contains quite high levels of oxalic acid.

SOUTHERNWOOD

Since very early times, southernwood (A*rtemisia abrotanum*) has been held in high regard for its medicinal, culinary and household uses. It was once known as 'old man' because it was thought to promote the growth of a new beard. Nicholas Culpeper wrote 'The ashes thereof, mingled with old sallet oyle, helps those what have their hair fallen and are bald causing their hair to grow again, either on the head or on the beard'. An infusion may be dabbed directly on to the scalp to ease irritations, flaking or dandruff. Use this recipe as a final rinse after shampooing. It will help to offset any scalp dryness or flyaway hair.

Tip:

Southernwood, with its lemony tang, is an invigorating bath herb.

SOUTHERNWOOD HAIR RINSE

3 *tablespoons southernwood*

1 *tablespoon clary sage oil*

250 *ml apple cider vinegar*

50 *ml whisky*

Combine all the ingredients in a lidded jar and steep for 2 weeks. Strain and rebottle.

SPEARMINT

Spearmint (*Mentha spicata*), perhaps the most fragrant and best known of all the mints, is believed to have been cultivated by the ancient Egyptians. The Greeks also used it, adding sprays to their bathwater in much the same way as we use essences, salts and oils today. The Romans used it to decorate their tables and to flavour food. Early herbalists recommended rubbing bee and wasp stings with spearmint leaves to reduce redness and inflammation. Spearmint water was used as a refreshing facial tonic and was put into smelling bottles to prevent swooning. Spearmint oil and essence are quite usual ingredients in toothpastes and mouthwashes. Spearmint was an important ingredient in many early tooth-cleansing preparations. Try this old recipe for a spearmint tooth powder. It will rid the teeth of harmful plaque and unsightly stains and will leave the mouth and breath smelling fresh and sweet.

Tip:

Add 1 or 2 drops of spearmint oil or concentrate to cotton balls and place amongst stored clothes.

SPEARMINT TOOTH POWDER

2 tablespoons fresh spearmint leaves
2 tablespoons fresh sage leaves
3 to 4 tablespoons sea salt

Put the ingredients in a bowl and, using a pestle or some other heavy, smooth tool, crush them all to a fine powder. Place the mixture in a warm oven. When it is well baked and fairly hard, remove and pulverise a second time. Store in an airtight container.

STEAM

Once a week (more frequently if time and energy permit), a good steaming for the skin is soothing and beneficial for total health. Historically, many herbs have been used to soothe and heal the skin. Indeed, many cosmetics now incorporate a wide variety of herbs for their beneficial effects. It would be a good idea for you to use a few herbs while enjoying the relaxing quality of a good steam. Of course, each herb has many properties that will specifically affect your skin and body.

To give your face a special treat, try steaming it and then applying a natural facial mask. These together will open the pores and release deeply embedded dirt and toxins that cause muddy-looking skin. They also stimulate circulation, giving your face a healthy glow.

Cleanse your face thoroughly, and gently massage your favourite nourishing cream into the skin. Then, put 2 cups of water into an enamel pan, heat and add 2 tablespoons of a herb of your choice — try aloe vera, lavender, lemon grass, thyme or parsley, to name a few! Pine needles, cedar chips and cut lemons are also good. Steam your face by arranging a makeshift tent (made of a towel or plastic tablecloth) over the pan and enjoy your steam bath for 10 minutes or so. Rinse your face with tepid water to remove the residue of cream, pat your face dry and, lastly, use a natural astringent such as witch hazel or rosewater to close the pores.

For cleansing and soothing inflamed or reddened skin: try chamomile, nettle, rosemary or marigold in your facial steam.

For healing: try comfrey or fennel.

To tauten flabby skin: try peppermint or elder flower.

Tip:

Steaming is also a tried-and-true natural remedy for a blocked nose or sinus trouble. Use fresh-smelling herbs such as rosemary and peppermint or a few drops of nature's antiseptic oils, tea tree or eucalyptus, in a steam bath and inhale to help clear a stuffed-up head.

STRAWBERRY

Both the fresh bright-looking fruit and the leaves of the strawberry plant have nutritional and medicinal uses.

Strawberry leaves were commonly included in restoratives and tonics and, combined with other herbs like tansy and mallow, were mentioned as a wash for skin complaints and as gargles for the gums. The berries are astringent and diuretic and an excellent source of vitamins A and C. In fact, they provide four times as much vitamin C per serving as oranges, along with some calcium, iron, phosphorus, thiamine, riboflavin and potassium. They are low in salt and are a fairly high source of dietary fibre. Due to their high tannin content (7 to 10 per cent), both raw strawberries and infusions from the plant's leaves make excellent bowel tonics. Strawberry extract or concentrated strawberry juice is sometimes available in health food stores and a dash added to chamomile tea will help to cleanse and tone the entire system.

Tip:
To whiten teeth and remove tartar, paint teeth with strawberry juice, leave on for 5 minutes and rinse with warm water.

Tip:
A cut strawberry rubbed over the face will whiten skin.

Strawberries are also noteworthy as a wholesome and refreshing natural cosmetic. Being mildly astringent, they can be used to cleanse and tone the skin. Chewing the leaves for bleeding gums is a remedy that goes back to the time of Jesus Christ. Sixteenth century herbalists credited various parts of the plant with benefits, ranging from whitening the teeth to relieving sore throats and removing freckles. During the Napoleonic era, Madame Tallien supposedly added strawberry juice from crushed berries to her bath in order to soften her skin.

Tip:
Fresh juice from strawberry pulp has a cooling effect on feverish patients. Chop berries roughly and whirl in a blender with a little purified water.

TANSY

Tansy (*Tanacetum vulgare*) has been cultivated since Saxon times for its many culinary and medicinal uses, primarily in stuffings or for seasoning meat. Before mint became popular as an accompaniment to roast lamb, tansy sauce was served. It was used to flavour cakes eaten at Easter. Tansy puddings were commonly eaten during spring, tansy wine was an old remedy for stomach troubles and tansy tea was regarded as a cure for rheumatism. There was also a traditional dish known as a 'tansy', which was a type of omelette that could be made as either sweet or savoury.

Tansy's antiseptic and insect-repelling properties make it a useful natural scent in the kitchen. For the same reason, it was once used widely as a strewing herb and great bunches were hung in larders or meat safes. Gather and dry the leaves and flowers and add to potpourri to deter lice, fleas and flies. Try tansy tea and tansy tea bags for their tonic and digestive properties. Also, try an infusion of tansy (made with milk, not water) to fade freckles. Tansy has a slight bleaching effect on the skin and acts as a tonic to brighten up sagging skin.

TARRAGON

Unlike most other herbs, whose origins stretch back many centuries, tarragon (*Artemisia dracunculus*) does not appear in any medical literature until Tudor times, when John Evelyn wrote that 'Tis highly cordial and friendly to the heart, head and liver'. It was also considered a cure for toothache and — presumably due to its 'warming' taste

> **Tip:**
>
> Tarragon vinegar is very easy to make. Place a few sprigs into a glass bottle and pour over good-quality nonacetic white wine vinegar. Cork and steep on a sunny windowsill. This vinegar is marvellous in salads, especially with corn and carrots. It is also a useful digestive aid. Take a teaspoon before and after meals if you are prone to indigestion with certain 'windy' foods, like cucumbers or fish.

— an aphrodisiac. Another old belief was that tarragon was a cure for the bites of venomous snakes, scorpions, insects — even dragons. In fact, tarragon's Latin name *dracunculus* means 'little dragon'.

Tarragon has potent digestive properties, explaining its appearance both in old herbal texts as a cure for colic and as an ingredient on the labels of modern preparations for indigestion and flatulence. The Roman naturalist Pliny wrote that tarragon prevented fatigue, perhaps the reason for the still-current practice of pilgrims placing a sprig in their shoes.

Tarragon contains an essential oil, eugenol, which is the same anaesthetising oil found in oil of cloves, explaining its traditional use in alleviating toothache. Intriguing new research points to the use of tarragon in heart health, as it seems to help prevent the artery-narrowing plaque deposits associated with strokes. Also, like many culinary herbs, tarragon is useful as a first aid dressing for small wounds and minor cuts as it has a slight antibacterial effect.

TEAS, REGULAR

Regular black or Indian tea contains tannin, which is a natural healing agent and protects the skin. Use a cup of strong warm tea (strained) in a bath to relieve sunburn, or apply to any area of skin so affected with a cotton ball.

TEAS, HERBAL

Avoid tea and coffee, especially in the evening — caffeine surging through your bloodstream will not induce a good night's sleep. Try herbal teas, which are soothing and strengthening to the nerves. Lime flower and chamomile are both very good, as is lettuce. Use the dark green outer leaves of a cos lettuce and simmer gently in water for 10 minutes before straining the liquid.

TEA TREE OIL

Minor cuts and grazes will benefit from a wash with this natural antiseptic oil, as will facial pimples and other skin problems. The bruised, pulped leaves of the tea tree plant (*Melaleuca alternifolia*) can even provide emergency dressings if you are out in the bush. Just as the Native Americans used aromatic twigs of dogwood for toothbrushes, so tea tree twigs sharpened to a slanted edge make a pleasant and effective alternative to a forgotten toothbrush on a bush weekend.

Soak gauze pads with either neat or diluted tea tree oil or with tea tree ointment and use as a dressing to soothe and help to clear up cuts that are taking a long while to heal. These dressings should be changed frequently and the wound exposed to the air as often as possible. If a cut refuses to heal or begins to suppurate, then an astringent wash of tea tree oil in witch hazel followed by a loose compress of antiseptic herbs should help. For those affected with candidiasis, a douche containing a combination of 250 ml warm water and 1 tablespoon of slippery elm powder will help; add 3 drops of tea-tree oil to the mixture to increase its germ-killing potency.

Tip:
Topical application of tea tree oil is excellent for clearing athlete's foot. The oil may also be added to a footbath and used daily for this unpleasant fungal infection.

One of the best natural antibacterial substances for use by acne sufferers is tea tree oil. A recent Australian study compared a 5 per cent tea tree oil gel with benzoyl peroxide (used in some commercial acne preparations) in treating acne. It found that over a 3-month period a tea tree oil gel was an effective alternative to the standard topical acne treatments and produced far less irritation to the skin.

THREE IN ONE

This aromatic herb (*Coleus amboinicus*), also known as five seasons herb, is much used as a condiment in South-East Asian cookery and also in parts of South America, where it is known as Puerto Rican oregano or Cuban oregano. Its sweet scent has meant that it has also been much used in natural beauty care preparations, most often as a scented hair rinse or an ingredient in shampoos or conditioners. Pulped, the fresh leaves make a useful poultice for insect bites and stings.

THUJA

Athlete's foot is a fungal infection encouraged by hot weather and moist skin. It is easily picked up and spread in communal gyms and swimming pools. Symptoms include itching and rashes, splitting and peeling of the skin between the toes and blisters under them.

Thuja (*Thuja occidentalis*) ointment is a natural herbal treatment for athlete's foot. Thuja is the North American yellow cedar and the Native Americans call it the 'tree of life'. It can be used for tropical ulcers, tinea and plantar warts. It can also be used as a fungicide wash to clean the shower if you suspect a fungus of lurking there.

Tip:
Add essential oil of thyme to warmed olive oil and use as a stimulating rub for hair and scalp problems; this natural remedy is particularly appropriate in cases of persistent dandruff and flaking scalp.

THYME

Most thyme species, especially common thyme (*Thymus vulgaris*), have a long history of being used in cookery as well as medicine. Like other aromatic herbs, thyme was once used as a meat preservative. It is one of the most important herbs in Mediterranean cookery, its warm and spicy flavour marrying particularly well with the garlic, onions and tomatoes used in the cuisine of this area. It is a quintessential 'summer herb', producing a stronger flavour in hot sun, the pungent oils being drawn out by the heat.

Thyme was often mentioned in early medical treatises as an antiseptic, a cough remedy and a digestive aid. Although you may not realise it, thyme is probably already present in your home medicine chest. The oil is an indispensable ingredient in such household staples as Vicks Vaporub and Listerine. Thyme is a strong and effective natural remedy because of its tonic and antiseptic qualities, and it is especially useful when made into a mouthwash or decongestant. An infusion of fresh or dried thyme is a good general tonic or it may be used to rinse wounds or scratches.

The Romans used thyme as a digestive aid and as a remedy for 'melancholy', or hangovers! Herbalist Nicolas Culpeper recommended thyme tea as 'a soveraigne remedy to stayeth the hicket [hiccups] and also to combat that troublesome complaint, the night-mare'. Thyme is probably most effective as a natural remedy for coughs and colds, bronchitis and flu. German research has found that inhalations of thyme oil have considerable benefit in loosening phlegm and relaxing the respiratory tract.

Tip:

Try using a thyme cleanser for troubled or acneous skin. Combine 2 tablespoons of whole milk with 2 tablespoons of strong thyme tea, adding enough cornflour to thicken to a creamy consistency. Spread onto affected area and allow to remain for up to 5 minutes. Rinse well and pat dry with a soft towel.

Thyme was once burned on chafing dishes, carried from room to room by early housekeepers, to fumigate and perfume the air. You might like to toss a handful of dried thyme onto the fire in winter to similarly freshen the room, or try burning fragrant oil of thyme in an incense burner.

TOMATO

Put slices of raw tomatoes (*Lycopersicon esculentum*) on your face and leave them for 10 to 15 minutes. Obviously you will have to lie down to do this! You should mash the tomatoes up a little bit because it's the pulp that actually works as a bracing skin tonic. Spread the pulp over the area where large pores or blackheads are. It may sound odd — and you certainly look odd while you are doing it — but there is nothing ridiculous about this natural remedy. Tomatoes, after all, contain certain minerals, vitamins and amino acids that have an astringent effect on the skin.

Or make a tomato face mask by blending together equal amounts of tomato juice and the pulp of a lemon. Splash the mixture on your face, paying particular attention to the greasy areas, leave for 15 minutes, then wash off with tepid water.

TRAGACANTH

Tragacanth (*Astragalus gummifer*) is an Asiatic plant which exudes a gum, also called tragacanth. This is used as the basis for many natural setting lotions and as an additive in certain hair conditioners.

VALERIAN

Sleep researchers at the Nestlé Research Laboratories in La Tour-de-Peilz, Switzerland, serve steaming cups of this age-old sleep inducer, *Valeriana officinalis*. British doctors during World War II used tinctures of this herb to calm the shattered nerves of bombing raid victims. In a recent US study of sleep-troubled men and women, valerian produced significant improvements in sleep quality. Improvements were most noticeable among irregular or poor sleepers. Valerian does not affect dream recall or cause morning-after drowsiness the way prescription sleeping pills and over-the-counter sleep aids would. Valerian is available in tonic or tablet forms; alternatively, you could take it as a tea, though the taste is too pungent for most people. Or try this recipe.

Tip:
Because of its soporific effects, valerian is ideal for including in evening baths.

VALERIAN TEA

2 *teaspoons valerian*

1 *teaspoon cider vinegar*

3 *teaspoons raw honey*

3 *teaspoons vodka (optional)*

Place all ingredients in a teapot and cover with boiling water. Leave to steep for at least 5 minutes before pouring.

VERVAIN

A good herb for a relaxing body treatment is vervain (*Verbena officinalis*). Using a bath bag filled with vervain or an infusion of this herb is one of the simplest, cheapest and easiest ways of pampering yourself and so supporting your natural good health. Combine vervain with lavender, peppermint or pine needles for a stimulating effect, or with yarrow, marigold flowers or St John's wort for healing cuts and abrasions.

VIETNAMESE MINT

Despite its name, this is not really a member of the mint family. Rather than having the cooling taste of mint, Vietnamese mint (*Polygonum odoratum*) is very hot indeed. Probably best known for its culinary properties, being much used in the cuisine of Thailand and other Asian countries to add a hot spicy flavour to a recipe, it also has usefulness as a natural remedy. In Asian medicine, Vietnamese mint is used as a diuretic and, by association, to reduce fever.

VIOLETS

Called amongst other things 'Kit-run-the-streets' and 'Three faces in one head', violets (*Viola odorata*) have been used for many medicinal purposes since the Middle Ages. In his famous 17th century *Herball*, Nicolas Culpeper wrote that 'A strong decoction or syrup of the flowers is an excellent remedy for venereal disease. The spirit is good for the convulsions of children and a remedy for falling sickness [epilepsy], inflammation of the lungs and breasts, pleurisy, scabs and itch.'

Although violets are certainly not used for venereal disease these days, you may find if you visit a modern-day herbalist that violet syrup is still used as a gargle or a laxative and a tea made from the flowers is thought to have a calming influence on asthma and whooping cough. Both the leaves and roots of this humble small plant have mild laxative properties, explaining why you may see it listed as an ingredient in natural products for treating constipation or even coughs and flu, in line with the natural health principle of expelling toxins from the body. If you want to try your hand at making your own home remedy, a decoction of 15 g finely chopped root and fresh leaves is a most efficient purgative and is also helpful to the kidneys.

A compress of violets was once thought to be useful for headaches and sleeplessness, and it is a popular ingredient in potpourri and 'sleep pillows' for this reason. Most intriguing — though as yet unsubstantiated — are claims from European alternative medicine journals which state that eating violet leaves somehow thwarts certain types of cancer.

Tip:

An infusion of violets is an excellent skin-freshening lotion. It is particularly useful as a tonic for dry skin. Place a handful of flowers in boiling water and infuse for 15 minutes. Strain and store in a clean lidded glass jar in the refrigerator. Use this also as a scented rinse for your hair.

VITAMIN A

Vitamin A is essential to the body in developing and maintaining healthy eyes, skin, hair, teeth and gums as well as various glands. By maintaining the integrity of mucous membranes, it is vital to all cells; vitamin A fights infections, allergies and pollutants and, being an antioxidant, may protect against cancer. Vitamin A is often called 'the skin vitamin' as it plays a direct role in the body's ability to remove dead skin cells. Insufficient vitamin A or malabsorption of the vitamin if your digestive system is not properly processing fats (vitamin A is a fat-soluble vitamin) may lead to dry, scaly-looking skin. As vitamin A is part of the body's nutritional ammunition to fight infection, vitamin A supplementation often helps with pimply blemishes.

Vitamin A and its precursor betacarotene have been shown to increase immunity in animals and humans. Improved antibody levels and cellular immunity are produced by supplementation with these nutrients. Even the international cancer societies and associations all now recommend a diet high in betacarotene — which is converted in the body to vitamin A — as a cancer preventive. Individuals who are deficient in vitamin A derived from animal sources, or betacarotene from plants, heal less efficiently and are more susceptible to infection. Diabetics cannot convert betacarotene to vitamin A and are very likely to be deficient in the vitamin.

A very dry scalp may be an indicator of vitamin A deficiency, in which case your face and other areas of your skin such as the legs may also be very dry and sensitive, or even a little itchy. Vitamin A can help prevent dryness, blemishes, large pores, roughness and scaliness. It treats rough, goose-bumpy skin, combats acne and prevents premature ageing, especially wrinkling caused by dryness. It can contribute to healthy, shiny, resilient hair and help keep nails strong and smooth with no peeling or ridging.

Food sources rich in vitamin A include whole milk, butter, some margarines, eggs, leafy green and yellow vegetables and fruits (especially apricots, broccoli and turnips), fish liver oils, liver and kidneys.

There are a number of cosmetic treatments available which contain vitamin A or betacarotene, as well as supplements. Skin creams enriched with vitamins A and D are thought to retard the skin's ageing process, especially when used in conjunction with a course of skin tablets which also contain vitamin A.

Attention should be paid to the delicate eye area, to combat dryness. Try piercing a vitamin A or even a cod liver oil capsule and delicately patting the rich oil around the eyes. Acne, which strikes at menopause as often as it does at puberty, can be improved tremendously by the use of supplemental vitamin A, which helps counteract the tendency of dead skin cells to stick together and form comedone plugs. The application of a cream containing vitamins A and D will help prevent scarring and aid rapid healing.

An old-fashioned honey and egg mask will nourish the skin and leave it beautifully smooth, due to its high content of essential oils and vitamin A. Mix 1 dessertspoon of pure honey and the beaten yolk of 1 egg. Spread on the face and leave for 15 minutes before washing off with tepid water. Massaging the neck with fresh cream, another rich source of vitamin A, will help keep wrinkles at bay, while juiced lettuce leaves — another surprising source of vitamin A — are an old-time beauty remedy for enlarged pores on the nose and chin.

VITAMIN B COMPLEX

The B group vitamins help liberate energy from food by promoting the proper use of carbohydrates, proteins and fats by the body. They are necessary for the proper functioning of the heart and nervous system and essential to the health of all tissues in the body. B group vitamins comprise the 'backbone' of health, energy, wellbeing and good looks.

Tip:

An increased intake of B group vitamins is recommended for fungal foot infections.

The B vitamins help nourish the skin, keeping it rosier, more glowing (by cooperating with the thyroid) and smoother. They prevent heavy creasing of the skin, counteract liver spots, help combat acne and smooth tension lines. They can also contribute to strong and healthy nails. B vitamins are natural tranquillisers, helping to reduce those antagonists to good looks: stress and strain.

They are destroyed by alcohol, the Pill, antacids, sugar, baking soda and tobacco. Overlong exposure to the sun will also deplete the body's stores of B vitamins. It is essential to take the vitamin B complex in a balanced form: taking one alone, such as vitamin B_6 or B_{12}, can

Tip:

Lips need moisturising and protecting just as regularly as the rest of your face. If they are excessively dry or chapped, or peel often, check your intake of foods containing the B group vitamins.

create a severe deficiency of all the other members of the vitamin B family.

The B vitamins also play an important role in maintaining the health and beauty of the hair. These vitamins are not stored in the body, so adequate amounts must be ingested daily. Some of the B vitamins are synthesised in the intestines by the bacteria that normally inhabit that area. Antibiotics and anti-infective substances taken over a long period of time will kill off normal (along with harmful) gut bacteria, so a vitamin B deficiency may develop. It is advisable to take your vitamin B complex preparation along with yoghurt or buttermilk, which contains *Lactobacillus acidophilus*, the bacteria normally present in the colon.

In most instances, one can safely take large amounts of the B vitamins. They are water soluble so the body eliminates what it doesn't use. According to the late Adelle Davis, noted nutritionist, men who become bald early may have unusually high requirements for several of the B vitamins.

Wholegrain breads and cereals, brewer's yeast, milk, yoghurt, legumes, liver, eggs, leafy green vegetables, lecithin, wheat germ, raisins and some nuts are all good sources of vitamin B.

VITAMIN C

Vitamin C can be described on a label as ascorbic acid, calcium ascorbate and sodium ascorbate or, quite often, as a combination of all three forms of supply.

Vitamin C augments the general health of bone, teeth, skin, blood vessels, cartilage and tendons. It is essential in the formation of collagen, the all-important protein that helps support the body's actual structure. Sufficient vitamin C in the diet will keep the collagen strong and elastic, which will result in a taut, smooth skin.

Collagen is the predominant protein of the skin's connective tissue — the protein of hydration, formation and retention. Several excellent cosmetics utilise collagen — known as 'native collagen' — which has been developed without resorting to animal tests.

Vitamin C strengthens the underlying skin tissues, making it firmer with less sagging. It contributes to smoothness of skin, as opposed to blotchiness. It helps prevent dermatitis, psoriasis and acne. It combats liver spots and averts ugly bruises. It also works to firm up 'bags' beneath the skin by keeping skin firm and resilient.

Vitamin C is destroyed by overcooking and freezing of food and is lost when cut fruits and vegetables are exposed to the air. It may not be correctly utilised by the body if the bioflavonoids (found in citrus pith and pulp, for instance) are not present. Air pollution, industrial toxins, smoking, alcohol, aspirin, anticoagulant drugs, antidepressants, diuretics and antibiotics will all deplete the body of vitamin C, as will a high fever or infection.

Vitamin C is found primarily in citrus and other fruits, such as pawpaw, melon and berries, tomatoes, capsicum, leafy green vegetables, especially parsley and cabbage, and potatoes.

An old-time trick for the eyelids is to take a slice of raw potato, press it over the eye area and leave for 15 minutes. An alternative compress may be made by soaking gauze in freshly squeezed orange or lemon juice — both are, of course, excellent sources of vitamin C, which has firming and bleaching properties when applied topically to the skin. Similarly, strawberry pulp may be used both as a whitening polish for the teeth and as a refining facial mask, as may slices of tomato.

VITAMIN D

Vitamin D helps the body use calcium and phosphorus properly. Vitamin D helps normal kidney function, heart action, the nervous system and blood clotting. It also helps prevent tooth decay and governs muscular action.

Vitamin D is crucial for correct tooth formation and bone growth, combats acne and is necessary for proper glandular function — thus affecting one's entire appearance.

Vitamin D is lost through overcooking of foods and it may not be correctly utilised by the body unless calcium is present. It is also destroyed by cortisone, antacids and mineral oil laxatives.

Whole milk, egg yolks and avocados are all good food sources of vitamin D.

VITAMIN E

Vitamin E helps in the formation and function of red blood cells, muscle and other tissues. An antioxidant, it protects against air pollutants and other free radicals and aids in preventing lung disease. By maintaining the integrity of cell membranes, it is essential for the health of the circulatory and reproductive organs.

Vitamin E contributes to vibrant, lustrous hair. Greasy hair goes with a greasy scalp and usually a greasy skin — particularly down the centre of the face. Overactive sebaceous glands may cause the skin lubricant, sebum, to be excreted to excess. More often than not, it is an increase in oestrogen levels that causes the glands to overproduce. Vitamin E helps to normalise oestrogen levels, so it may be the most important beauty supplement of all. Acne and dandruff sufferers may also benefit by supplementing natural sources of vitamin E with vitamin E capsules or tablets.

By aiding the transport of fresh oxygen to the tissues, Vitamin E can also help tired skin look fresher. It helps replace moisture lost by the skin and arrests the ageing process. It wards off liver spots and is significant in varicose vein treatment. Vitamin E also checks lines under the eyes and on the lips and is unparalleled in diminishing topical skin scarring.

Vitamin E also helps the body respond to stress and is effective for premenstrual and menopausal tension. It improves circulation and heals skin ulcers, bed sores, burns and scars.

Antagonists to vitamin E include oxidising agents used in food processing, rancid fats and oils, supplementation with inorganic iron, the Pill and mineral oil laxatives. X-rays and excessive sugar intake are also thought to damage vitamin E in the body.

Vegetable oils, wholegrain cereals, brown rice, wheat germ, lettuce, asparagus, broccoli, cabbage, yeast, nuts, eggs, molasses and sweet potatoes are all rich in vitamin E.

Many natural beauty products contain extra vitamin E for its smoothing and moisturising properties. Vitamin E may be added to any face or hair product with great benefit. Both vitamin E concentrate (capsules or ampoules are good) and wheat germ oil are excellent conditioners for the skin and hair, either added to shampoo or applied directly. For skin moisturising, whisk together 1 tablespoon of wheat germ oil with liquid vitamin E, or use it alone.

Tip:

An instant hair revitaliser that will restore sheen and relieve dry, itchy scalps is vitamin E. Prick one or two capsules and rub the contents directly onto your hair at the roots, then comb it through, making sure it reaches the ends. If your hair doesn't look too oily, leave it in till the next shampooing.

WALNUT

Long used as a natural dye for wool by craftspeople, walnut skins have a positive benefit as a natural cosmetic, and may be used to darken hair.

Combine 6 tablespoons chopped green walnut skins with 1 tablespoon alum powder (from the chemist). Add a little warm water, just enough to make a paste, and rub evenly through hair. Leave for approximately 1 hour, then rinse off and shampoo with a mild shampoo.

Tip:

An infusion of walnut leaves added to a bath will soothe the nerves and help to promote sleep.

WATER

Water is an essential ingredient in many natural remedies and cosmetic preparations. When making any of the recipes mentioned in this book, remember that they will keep longer if distilled or purified water is used. Spring water or rainwater is good for the complexion and hair; to 'soften' tap water, leave it in an uncovered jug overnight.

Don't forget your inner health, either! Drink large amounts of cool water on hot days. Avoid heavily iced drinks and alcoholic beverages. Next most important after fresh water are unsweetened fruit juices, particularly delicious tropical fruit juices. Pineapple, pawpaw, mango and passionfruit are all rich in vitamins A and C, which are excellent for nourishing the skin.

WATERCRESS

Watercress (*Nasturtium officinale*) is a delicious and refreshing herb, much used as a condiment and a 'salading' since the Middle Ages. Its name is a direct reference to its preferred growth habit — it does best in fresh running water, especially where the nearby soil has a high lime content. Watercress may be used in soups and mixed green salads, adding a refreshing peppery taste. It is also available in tablet and tonic form.

An old German saying, which roughly translates as 'Eat cress!', was once applied to patients thought to have lost their memory. Indeed, being very high in vitamin C and iron, watercress is a valuable tonic herb and digestive for elderly people, so it could have the effect of 'perking up' a lethargic patient. The Persians were said to have dosed their children with watercress, much as we would have used cod liver oil, to improve their strength and health. During the 17th century, watercress was used both as an antiscorbutic (to counter scurvy) and, pulped, as a cleansing poultice for those troubled with pimples.

Sixteenth century herbalist John Gerard recommended watercress leaves be used 'by young maids to keep their complexions faire'. And 17th century herbalist Nicolas Culpeper gave a recipe for 'Cresses Water': 'The leaves bruised or the juice is good to be applied to the face or other parts troubled with freckles, pimples, spots, or the like, at night, and washed away in the morning'. As watercress also contains a good supply of sulphur, it certainly would have had value as an anti-acne herb. Its diuretic properties would also have advantages in treating this condition, by helping to flush out wastes and toxins which may be causing an internal imbalance manifested in the pimples.

Tip:
If using fresh watercress, select the fresh new leaves rather than the older ones, which have a tougher texture and less pleasant taste.

Tip:
For a natural aid to tone down freckles, combine the juice of a bunch of water-cress with 1 teaspoon of honey and apply as a bleaching mask. Rinse off after 5 to 7 minutes.

WHEAT GERM

To soften extra-hard skin, such as on the elbows, knees, soles of the feet or backs of the heels, mix up equal quantities of wheat germ oil and lemon juice and massage in. Alternatively, use equal quantities of wheat germ oil and apple cider vinegar. Keep rubbing in until all the oil is absorbed.

Dry skin responds particularly well to wheat germ. To make a rich facial moisturising treatment, combine 1 egg yolk with 1 teaspoon of wheat germ and enough almond oil to form a paste. Warm slightly if desired and spread over the face, or brush on with a cosmetic brush. Leave for 10 to 15 minutes, then rinse off with tepid water and pat dry with a soft towel.

Tip:
For cracked, dry toenails, rub wheat germ oil into the nail bed each night.

WINTERGREEN

Synthetic oil of wintergreen can be added to a carrier oil, such as olive or fine almond oil, and used as a soothing rub for athletic injuries which involve twisting of joints and stretched, sprained or torn connective tissues. Natural wintergreen or deerberry (*Gaultheria procumbens*) is probably too strong, although the warmed, pulped leaves can be used as a poultice. Natural oil of wintergreen was once used as a base for the commercial preparation of aspirin as it contains menthyl salicylate. Along the same lines, an infusion of the leaves may be used as a natural remedy for a headache; it is also useful as a mouthwash for sore throats and inflamed gums, as a compress for skin problems and in a poultice to relieve the pain of rheumatism.

WITCH HAZEL

The bark and twigs of the witch hazel shrub (*Hamamelis virginiana*) are used to make a styptic, antiseptic and cleansing lotion. It is high in tannic acid, an astringent which is both soothing and refreshing, and can help reduce the size of broken capillaries.

Use the pure extract as a soothing compress for rashes and bites, or combine with comfrey ointment as a poultice for varicose veins. For the complexion, diluted witch hazel should be dabbed on with a moistened cotton ball after cleansing with a pure gentle soap such as Castile. Blisters may be treated with iced witch hazel. A wash made from witch hazel extract or leaves bound loosely in a compress will help both to soothe and to heal broken blisters and abrasions. Witch hazel, with its powerful astringent and styptic effects, is a common ingredient in natural products for treating haemorrhoids, skin irritations, sunburn, insect bites, varicose veins and tired feet. A herbalist may prescribe witch hazel for internal use, too, to treat diarrhoea or excessive menstrual flow and internal bleeding.

Tip:

Rub the soles of aching feet with witch hazel and lemon juice to get the circulation going. Athletes could try massaging a liquid made of witch hazel, rosewater and violet oil into their overworked feet to relieve strain and soothe sore muscles. A mixture of witch hazel with 4 drops of clove oil is another tonic for aching feet.

Try a refreshing witch hazel facial 'steam' — combine equal parts of witch hazel, lemon grass and lavender, and gently simmer for 5 minutes. Stand over steam with a towel draped over your head for 10 minutes to open the pores and increase circulation. Then splash skin with a chilled tonic of diluted witch hazel and vinegar.

A most effective mouthwash for bleeding gums can be made by grinding up 3 tablespoons of the tannin-rich witch hazel leaves and adding them to 1 litre of boiling water. Then strain the liquid through fine muslin. When cool, rinse the preparation through the mouth three times a day.

YARROW

Yarrow (A*chillea millefolium*) has a penetrating odour when it is brushed against or crushed in the fingers. It is named for the Greek god Achilles, who was taught the plant's medicinal benefits by the centaur Chiron. Yarrow is native to the British Isles and was much used there by mediaeval 'herb wyfes' for its healing effects.

Yarrow tea may be drunk to soothe a sore throat and yarrow essence or dried powdered yarrow are both ingredients in demulcent tonics to soothe the throat and gastrointestinal tract, and in certain cosmetics. In France, yarrow was once known as 'l'herbe aux charpentiers' because it was used to heal wounds caused by the carpenter's tools. A tea made from yarrow may be used as a tonic to neutralise greasy skins; it is also a hair tonic.

Tip:

The ancient Chinese valued yarrow for its astringent and relaxing properties. When infused in bathwater, it will help to soothe muscular aches and pain.

YEAST, BREWER'S

While the excellent nutritional properties of yeast — in beer and bread, for instance — were recognised early, the identification of various factors which cured deficiency diseases did not occur until the early part of this century. In particular, the B complex vitamins were recognised and identified, and several of them were first extracted from yeast. The more important ones are biotin, nicotinic acid, pantothenic acid, folic acid, pyridoxine, riboflavin and thiamine.

A nutritional yeast supplement, such as brewer's yeast to which no additional vitamins have been added, contains approximately the following amounts of B complex vitamins (in micrograms per gram): thiamine (B_1), 60–100; riboflavin

Tip:

A supplement of brewer's yeast tablets and large helpings of wheat germ are recommended for anyone with a hair problem. It has also been said that grey hair can be helped by large doses of brewer's yeast.

(B_3), 35–50; niacin, 300–500; biotin, 1–2; pyridoxine, 25–30; pantothenic acid, 70; and folic acid, 5–13. Brewer's yeast contains negligible amounts of sodium and is an excellent source of potassium, phosphorus and other minerals. Yeast products supply many valuable trace minerals, among them copper, selenium, manganese, chromium, molybdenum, zinc, silicon and sulphur.

Tip:

Brewer's yeast makes an invigorating facial tonic. Combine 1 teaspoon of powdered brewer's yeast with enough warm water to form a paste, and apply to facial skin as a mask. Allow to dry, then rinse off and pat dry with a soft towel.

Brewer's yeast, sprinkled over cereal or added to freshly squeezed juice, is my preferred way of ensuring an adequate intake of B group vitamins. A tasty alternative to tablets or powder is some of the savoury yeast-based spreads you will find in your health food store or the natural foods sections of supermarkets; several brands of nerve tonics also include brewer's yeast, as do some of the cereal beverages.

Tip:

Brewer's yeast is an antidote for sunburn, should you be foolish enough to let this happen to you. Break up a cake of yeast — or crush 5 tablets — mix with ½ cup of cider vinegar and blend well. This has a noticeably cooling effect on the skin.

You can mix brewer's yeast powder with honey (or witch hazel or wheat germ oil) and an egg and apply as a toning, regenerative mask. As with the B group vitamins, brewer's yeast is a valuable supplement for the hair, helping to enhance and preserve your crowning glory.

YOGHURT

Yoghurt will soften dry skin. Stir 1 teaspoon of malt vinegar into a small carton of natural yoghurt. Brush mixture all over the feet: soles, heels and between the toes. Leave for 5 minutes, then rinse off and pat dry. Yoghurt can also be very beneficial as a treatment for oily skin. Combine 3 tablespoons of yoghurt with 1 tablespoon of brewer's yeast and 2 teaspoons of lemon juice. This will make a liquid facial formula which can be easily brushed onto the skin and allowed to dry for 10 to 15 minutes, then rinsed off.

ZINC

Zinc deficiency has been found to be the culprit in many cases of hair loss. In food processing and refining, zinc is lost and not replaced. For example, whole-wheat flour contains almost four times the zinc found in processed white flour. Cooking destroys over 40 per cent of the zinc in spinach and over 80 per cent in tomatoes. A nutritional deficiency of zinc is also sometimes related to an excess of copper in your environment, such as copper hot water services (instead of the old zinc-in-galvanised-iron pipes), or to contraceptive devices or a number of other causes. Zinc is also an important micronutrient in the male hormonal pattern.

A change of diet to one composed of natural, unprocessed food will supply zinc. Nuts, seeds, seafood and wholegrain products are all good sources of zinc. Certain foods are especially high in zinc, such as peanuts and peanut butter, so if you have a craving, this may be the reason! If zinc supplements are necessary, have a doctor or nutritionist recommend the optimum dosage for your height, age and weight.

Supplemental zinc has also been shown to be useful in the treatment of acne. Scientific studies show that supplemental zinc increases the body's utilisation of vitamin A, the 'skin vitamin'. Supplemental vitamin A seems to help by counteracting the tendency of dead skin cells to stick together and form comedone plugs, leading to infection, inflammation and blackheads. Take a minimum of 30 mg of zinc daily for 3 months and 10 to 30 mg thereafter. Since vitamin A and zinc work so well together, it is only logical that both be taken simultaneously for optimum benefit.

INDEX TO DISORDERS

abscesses 129
aching joints 18, 24, 138
    see also arthritis;
    rheumatism
aching muscles 24
acne
    dietary treatment 163,
    166, 167, 170, 176
    topical treatment 21,
    97, 116, 156
age spots 139, 166, 168
anaemia 125
anaesthetics 3
antibiotics 14, 48, 66, 116
antidepressants 29, 51, 63,
    102, 122, 135
antihistamines 74
anti-inflammatories
    see inflammation
antiperspirant 141
antiseptics 36, 48, 68, 93,
    102, 129, 158
antispasmodics 25, 50
anxiety 123
aromatherapy 67-8
arrhythmia 31, 83, 102
arteries, hardening of 31
arthritis 18, 24, 42, 69
asthma 68, 161
athlete's foot 9, 157
athletic injuries 11, 55, 171

bad breath 45, 138
baldness 92-3
    see also hair loss
bed-wetting 142
bee stings 127
biliary duct disorders 6
bladder disorders 6, 20,
    150
blisters 57
blood pressure 19, 26
    high 31, 58, 83
    low 31
blood purifiers 29, 66, 141
blood vessels strengthener
    31
blotches 54
boils 74, 129
bowel
    disorders 30, 121
    inflammation 19
    tonics 153
breast milk production 73
bronchitis 54, 59, 68, 158
bruises

around the eye 149
compresses and poul-
    tices 11, 34, 37, 46, 55,
    61
dressing 125
gel 75
rub 18, 36
burns 75, 97

candida 90
candidiasis 1, 78, 156
capillaries
    broken 172
    surface 23
catarrh 81
chapping 97
chilblains 31
childbirth 96, 134
cholesterol 98
circulation
    aid 91
    disorders 83
    stimulants 41, 79, 107,
    117, 138-9
cold sores 54
colds 27, 74, 158
colic 9, 36, 37, 41, 44, 56-7,
    72, 80, 103, 106, 118, 128,
    155
constipation
    dietary aids 1, 46, 61, 130
    prevention *see* laxatives
contact rashes 9
coughs 27, 54, 67, 68, 114,
    122, 158
    see also decongestants
cracked skin 9
cramps 25, 50
    see also menstrual cramps
cystitis *see* urinary tract
    infections

dandruff 9, 23, 92-3, 139,
    167
dead skin cells 11, 70, 162,
    176
decongestants 87, 128, 138,
    142, 158
deodorant 141
depression 29, 51, 63, 102,
    122, 135
dermatitis 9, 23, 166
diarrhoea 3, 22, 38, 50, 51,
    61, 65, 73, 86, 149
digestive aids
    dietary fibre 30, 119

edible 8, 64-5, 72-3,
    77-8, 126
    infusions 56, 72-3, 105
    oils 3, 15, 39, 86
    teas 15, 22, 96, 108,
    111, 117-18, 127, 138,
    144-5, 154
    tonics 42-3, 104, 170
digestive problems 36, 40,
    44, 101
    see also indigestion
diuretics 37-8, 42, 51, 58,
    59, 63, 67, 88, 93, 102,
    125, 161, 170
diverticulitis 30
dizziness 80
douche 1, 96
dry hair 12
    see also hair care
dry skin 4, 12, 53, 55, 79,
    111, 119, 122, 163, 171, 174
    see also skin care
feet 4, 145
dyspepsia *see* indigestion

earache 113
eczema 12, 117
exhaustion 129
eyes, inflamed 25, 46-7, 58,
    71, 73, 81, 136

fever 10, 14, 26, 28, 32, 40,
    45, 51, 66, 74, 86, 99, 111,
    135, 141
flatulence 3, 36, 37, 41, 50,
    56, 65, 73, 80, 128, 155
fleas 3, 126-7, 154
flu 158
fluid replacement 27
fluid retention 63, 67
    see also diuretics
footbaths 55, 99, 145
forgetfulness 48
fungal infections 9, 35-6,
    114, 157

gallstones 63
gastrointestinal problems
    2
gout 43, 63, 117
grazes 125
gums, inflamed 23, 171
gynaecological complaints
    25-6, 27, 134
    see also menstrual flow;
    uterus

haemorrhoids 40, 42, 75, 86
hair care 4, 7-8, 10, 32,
39-40, 44-5, 49-50, 52, 87,
121-4
hair loss 23, 176
see also baldness
hardening of the arteries 31
head colds 27
headaches 4, 18, 74, 98,
102, 138, 141, 171
migraines 22
heart disorders
arrythmias 31, 83, 102
palpitations 31, 48, 113
tachycardia 113
heartburn 6, 80
herpes simplex 90
hyperacidity 111
hysteria 74

immune system boosters
66, 69, 146, 162-3
indigestion 2, 3, 41, 50, 56,
58, 73, 155
see also digestive aids;
digestive problems
inflammation 75
anti-inflammatories 46,
51
bowels 19
eyes 25, 46-7, 58, 71, 73,
81, 136
gums 23, 171
intestines 109
skin *see* skin, inflamed
throats 67, 89, 108, 114,
171, 173
influenza 158
insects
bites 35, 36, 58, 74, 88,
125, 157
repellents 126-7, 127,
154
stings 127, 157
insomnia *see* sleeplessness

joint pains *see* aching joints

kidney disorders 6, 20, 93,
125, 150

laxatives 2, 38, 39, 47, 51,
76, 104, 121, 131-2, 161
lice 3
liver complaints 32
liver spots 139, 166, 168

masks 109-10, 119-20, 164

menopausal tension 168
menstrual cramps 9, 25-6,
44, 80, 107, 108, 136
menstrual flow, excessive
19, 27, 96, 99
migraines 22
see also headaches
mouth
infections 24-5
sores 114
ulcers 74, 81
muscles, aching 24

nappy rash 54
nausea 50, 56, 59, 101
see also vomiting
nervous exhaustion 119,
142
nervous tension 40
neuralgia 4, 114

oedema 58
oily skin 82, 96, 97, 101,
173

palpitations 31, 48, 113
perspiration 141
pimples 36, 54, 97-8
PMT 25-6, 69, 168
pregnancy 112
see also childbirth
premenstrual syndrome
25-6, 69, 168
psoriasis 166

rashes 54
respiratory tract infections
40
rheumatism
dietary aids 43, 63, 67
muscular 26
topical treatment 3, 18,
20, 24, 36, 114, 171

scabies 3
sciatica 114
seborrhoea 23
sedatives 25, 44, 59, 86, 123,
135, 164
sinus-related complaints
87
see also decongestants
skin
see also skin care
cracked 9
disorders 2, 69, 81
eruptions 7, 85
inflamed 59, 88, 139

preservation 85, 99-100,
136-7
softeners 81
stretched 42
tonics 10, 49, 61, 96,
101, 116, 130, 136, 159
skin care 32-3, 88, 123, 153
see also dry skin; oily skin
dead skin cells 11, 70,
162, 176
facial 128
ingrained dirt 147
oils 120-1
steaming 151-2, 172
sleeplessness 40, 65, 74,
86, 101, 103, 119, 122-3,
135, 160
spasms *see* cramps
splinters 2
sports injuries 11, 55, 171
sprains 1, 36, 75, 131
compresses and poul-
tices 11, 37, 46, 79, 122
stimulants 58
stings 127, 157
stomach complaints 32, 65
sunburn 57, 97, 155
sunscreens 147
swellings 55, 61, 75, 81

tachycardia 113
temperature imbalances 80
throats, inflamed 67, 89,
108, 114, 171, 173
thyroid activity, low 94
tinea 9, 157
tonsillitis 24, 26-7
toothache 4, 37, 52, 101,
115, 155
tranquillisers *see* sedatives

urinary tract infections 58-9,
60, 63, 65, 67, 78, 109, 111
uterus
discharge 19
stimulant 42

varicose conditions 23, 86,
168, 172
vomiting 52
see also nausea

wasp stings 127
whooping cough 161
wounds 61
dressing 106, 122, 135,
149
washing 1-2